Lois,

I am always grateful for our friendship and your generous support. Will talk to you soon.

Love,
Carole

Playing the Game of Life on God's Turf

Other title by the author:

Bunkie Emeritus: Climbing Up the Downside of Dementia with My Mom

Playing the Game of Life on God's Turf

Carole Cash Stemley

VANTAGE PRESS
New York

FIRST EDITION

Copyright © 2006 by Carole Cash Stemley

Published by Vantage Press, Inc.
419 Park Ave. South, New York, NY 10016

Manufactured in the United States of America
ISBN: 0-533-15205-4

Library of Congress Catalog Card No.: 2005902684

0 9 8 7 6 5 4 3 2 1

To the spirit of two pioneers in my life
who taught me to play **the game** by
the examples of their lives:

My mother,
Carrie Mae Grove
(1913–2000),

and grandmother,
Lola Mae Starks Grove
(1897–1984)

**To God be the glory
for His unchanging hand of love
and faithfulness.**

Contents

Acknowledgments

I am especially grateful to the following "home team players" for their gracious and invaluable involvement in the completion of this book: Dr. and Mrs. Thomas E. Adger, Mrs. Louise Gaddy, Mr. Raymond Gambrell, Mrs. Fredericka Hurley, Mrs. Mary E. Kendrick, Bishop and Mrs. Nathaniel Linsey, Ms. Monique Prather, Mrs. Virginia Prather, and Mr. and Mrs. Thomas E. Wood, Jr.

Pre-Game Commentary

Life is huge because of God and not always fair because of us. In addition to the air we breathe, the color of our skin, and all of what we see and do, life is each of us and everything that makes us alike and different; it's the entire human experience. More in keeping with the contents of this book, life is a two-fold effort of faith and pressing on to the state of perfection that exists only in eternity with God.

Our minute-to-minute behavior within and outside that effort accounts for life being the greatest game played this side of heaven. From the moment God created man, the game of life has since begun with every birth and with the hands of time already in motion as the manager of change.

Time is the supreme clock of life that ends yesterday and begins tomorrow. Each new day advances us to another time frame of life and, at the very least, causes us to reflect on one of our yesterdays. Memories of the past often remind us of how things were at other times in our private lives and with the way of the world.

As the guardian of our destiny, time separates childhood from adolescence and adolescence from adulthood. Along with our physical growth at various stages of life, we are expected to show higher levels of maturity in our personal and social conduct. Many times, any opportunity for us to experience the "abundant life" depends on our pace and level of maturity. Whereas our ability to manage life improves with experience, progressive maturity is far more beneficial to our ability to manage change.

For better or worse, life is flooded with change. As the one constant motion of life, change is our appointment with destiny. The longer we live individually or endure as a society, the longer we face change as a way of life and make choices according to our character and circumstances.

The world has shown enormous strength in changing its ancient cradle of civilization. In the race of technology, American society has come a long way from its days of the pony express. Change in our social values, standards of acceptable behavior, and moral conscience is no less apparent. Yet, as the saying implies, the more we change, the more we stay the same. And so it is with God's turf and the game of life that He allows us to play with an unrestricted freedom of choice.

On yesterday, the Garden of Eden was a land of beauty with an original cast of four characters that included the devil as God's main opponent. Today, that same beautiful garden includes our homes, churches, schools, government buildings, shopping malls, abortion clinics, hotels, night clubs, beauty salons, prisons, drug rehabilitation centers, and a massive population of diverse game players. But the garden is still God's turf. Furthermore, the rules of the game and the characters remain unchanged.

As it is with any game, the intended goal may or may not be accomplished. Though our gains may offset our losses at different intervals of the play period, the game never ends with a tied score. Once we reach the finish line, we either win or lose.

On God's Turf is a personal approach to life as a game, with emphasis on social change and circumstances. In addition to establishing various aspects of the game and detailing some of the moves that we make, attention is also given to why the winners and losers will always be the same.

Playing the Game of Life
on God's Turf

What Was God Thinking?
(Biblical Foundations of the Game)

Life became more than just a dream on the day of Adam and Eve's eviction from the Garden of Eden. It began as a gift of God's breath in His creation of mankind. But, for ages of time, that same gift has been wrapped by the hands of society with a price tag. Since we no longer live free of charge, life for many in today's world is little more than the hustle and bustle of a work week or the long wait for retirement. Though work is an inherited routine of survival, the human experience generally provides a greater field of activity from which we develop our regard for life.

Our outlook on life either stabilizes or changes from time to time because of personal and social experiences. Regardless of how consistent or flexible our views may be, life is always a matter of personal perspective. One person's joy can easily be another person's sorrow.

Our regard for life is further limited or extended on the basis of our attitudes, skills, and resources. Life, then, for some of us is as simple as eating a piece of chocolate cake, while for others it's a hardship that can be more challenging than climbing Mount Everest without a rope. Yet, from another perspective, life can be as broad as the difference between freedom and slavery, or as thin as the line between love and hate.

Any attempt to restrict human life to a single concept would also prove frail and improper because each of us

1

contributes a distinct presence or quality to the world, even as a mere add-on to the census bureau count. On this basis, perhaps life can be appropriately declared as our purpose on earth, the natural aspects of which include our obligation to society, community service, responsibility to family, self-preservation, and obedience to God. Whether our purpose is active, idle, or even godly, all that we do or fail to do in support of our purpose becomes the game of life that we play on the many stages of God's turf.

Playing the game of life is a full-time activity that combines the private and public agenda of our thoughts, words, and deeds. Each move that we make in the game defines who we are in relationship to God and to our fellow man. This feature alone is sufficient in making the game of life unlike any other game played on earth, but there are other features that are equally significant.

In contrast to championship games that are sponsored by major associations and leagues of organized sports, the game of life is the Super Bowl of all sports. It's the ultimate championship game that differs from the world of organized sports in several respects, beginning with the rules that actually define the goal and players of the game.

Rules are so much a part of the American way that we have rules for making rules. Between the United States Constitution and family curfews, rules are necessary for maintaining social order and a sense of human decency. They set the standards by which we live, learn, play, work, and worship together or individually at all social levels. Rules also set the standards by which we are punished. But as the world changes, so do the rules of man. The same principle applies when the situation is reversed; new rules change the way of the world.

Unfortunately, all rules are not good rules. We have

witnessed and have been victimized by negative effects of many rules that once legalized or tolerated wrongful practices. In fact, the need to change or abolish such rules has resulted in many historical events that shattered the status quo. Otherwise, barriers of "colored water" and the Iron Curtain would be the rule of the day. The notion, however, that rules are made to be broken is quite dangerous whenever it is stated without exceptions.

The governance of human life is God's business. Whether created in times of social harmony or civil unrest, rules that are designed by man for the governance of man are likely to be modified in some way. But there are rules other than those made by man that are the exception because they are permanent and have total dominion over mankind. They are the rules of God that people around the world, despite their personal convictions and religious faith, recognize as the Ten Commandments. These rules are the same now as they were when given to Moses by God for the people of Israel and for all future generations of the world.

The significance of the Ten Commandments to the Biblical foundation of our lives justifies applying them as the rules of the game.

Thou shalt have no other God before me. Thou shalt not make unto thee any graven image, or any likeness of anything that is in the heaven above, or that is in the earth beneath, or that is in the water under the earth. . . . Thou shalt not take the name of the Lord thy God in vain. . . . Remember the Sabbath day, to keep it holy. Honour thy father and thy mother. . . . Thou shalt not kill. Thou shalt not commit adultery. Thou shalt not steal. Thou shalt not bear false witness against thy neighbor. Thou shalt not covet thy neighbour's house, thou shalt not covet thy neighbour's wife, nor his manservant, nor his maidservant, nor his ox, nor his ass, nor anything that is thy neighbour's.[1]

Familiarity with God's Commandments usually begins in bits and pieces during our early childhood years. Upon completing in-house boot camp training for tots, some of us may have been stage-struck performers or stage-frightened victims who were coached into finishing a bashful, if not teary recitation of "honor thy father and thy mother." This is the lead speech for toddlers on Mother's Day and Father's Day programs.

Aside from coaxing their young into disastrous performances, parents usually have to caution their toddlers against taking other folks's property without permission. Children are also generally taught to love God and to tell the truth. In instances such as these, whether intended or not, at least some of God's rules are being taught, learned, memorized, and practiced.

Departure from childhood seems to be a main turning point in the human emphasis on doing the right thing according to God. The focus of that particular effort tends to shift more toward the human domain of satisfying personal goals and interests. Eventually, there is contentment in following the crowd at the cost of dismissing godly principles or independently staging personal acts of moral compromise. Just as drivers exceed speed limits, hoping not to be seen or stopped by a traffic cop, we break the Commandments of God with the hope that He neither sees nor hears us. Least of all do we think that God would actually stop us on the spot. Many times, because we deny or simply ignore the omnipotence of God's presence, He is nowhere in our hopes or thoughts.

A natural aspect of the game, then, is our tendency to break the rules of God quicker and much more frequently than we ever think about breaking the rules of man. Given half a chance, we sometimes try to justify wrong until we either believe or can convince others that wrong is right. Yet, with all of the misdeeds that we commit against God and against each other, God loves us anyway and forgives us as we forgive each other.[2] God's love for us is not our only security in the game. Our survival in life is also based on His grace and mercy.

God specifically grants us a lifetime margin of human error that expands our purpose on earth to include righting our wrongs. Such a step is the pure art of penitence, but the art of playing the game of life on God's turf involves much more effort. Victory hinges on a number of other requirements set by God.

Everything that needs to be known about man's purpose in relationship to God is revealed by the Word of God in the Holy Bible. The Ten Commandments provide the full scope of our purpose, which is to love and honor God with obedience. Constant pursuit of that purpose is the ideal way to win the game. Unfortunately, along the route of human pursuit, we take temporary rest periods by the wayside day after day, month after month, and year after year.

Our stop and go efforts in honoring and obeying God are not incidental. Before the time of human existence, God knew that we would break His laws. The fact that He created us anyway makes it easy to wonder, "What was God thinking?" The answer is ageless because it begins and ends with God.

God's perfection as creator and ruler of earth is absolute.[3] Everything that He does is, therefore, perfect according to His plan; **not ours.** Furthermore, man's failure to keep God's Commandments is even perfect, but only according to God's plan. Clarification of that opinion is presented in other sections of this book. The more immediate and important point is that God deliberately loves each of us so much that He compensates for our weakness.

The full package of God's creation includes a prominent and everlasting gift for all mankind. The provision of that gift was foretold by prophets centuries before becoming a reality: "Behold a virgin shall conceive, and bear a son, and shall call His name Immanuel."[4] In God's own time, barely two thousand years ago, He fulfilled that prophecy with the birth of His Son, Jesus Christ.

Jesus walked among men on earth as "the way, the truth, and the life."[5] During the time between His manger and a rugged cross, Jesus enhanced man's purpose on earth in several ways. He taught us how to live by the example of His life and by principles based on the laws of God. His death was our past, present, and future guarantee of salvation because, in the crucifixion of Christ, God settled the score of our sins forever. Finally, the resurrection of Jesus from the dead confirmed the spirit of a living God and His offer of eternal life to us.

Whereas God gave His Son to the world as a gift with no strings attached, reaping the full benefits of that gift presents a different situation altogether. Any chance that we may have to receive the championship prize of eternal life requires us to believe in Jesus as the Son of God, and to accept Him as our personal Saviour. Otherwise, we perish.[6] Among other requirements, we must also repent for all of our sins.[7]

Common knowledge of heaven and hell leads us to believe that people really want to go to heaven when they die. That belief not only reflects worldly thought, it's the universal hope among all Christians. However, the caution from an old and notable Negro spiritual warns that, "ev'rybody talkin' 'bout heav'n ain't goin' there." The message of this song implicates one of the basic principles that Jesus taught, "Not everyone that saith unto me Lord, Lord, shall enter the kingdom of heaven."[8] This principle, alone, clearly extends our requirements beyond that of having faith in God.

The honor of going to heaven is also bestowed on the basis of our self-worth while on earth. This condition indicates the need for us to work our souls into heaven because all faith and no work makes any heaven-bound aspiration null and void.[9] The overall goal in the game, then, is to prove our faith by our deeds. In conjunction with making preparations for an upward journey, the Holy Bible is the most adequate source of information available on the international market.

Man has historically relied on the Bible for a variety of reasons that relate to life and living. It excels and overpowers any other sense of direction that we may have from and to God. Because of its dynamic impact on the human experience, the Bible is selected as the "players' manual" for the game of life. In addition to providing all of the rules and moves that we need to be aware of as players, the Bible clarifies our entire relationship to God in many of its passages.

As a book of proof, the Bible documents all of God's properties in an unmistakable summary, "The earth is the Lord's, and the fullness thereof; the world, and they that dwell therein."[10] Given that clarity of ownership, until earth is advertised, "For Sale," by God, it is His turf and we are His people.[11]

From an athletic point of view, the whole world is God's grand sports arena where every living person plays the game of life; from the youngest to the oldest, the smallest to the biggest, the poorest to the richest, the sickest to the healthiest, the most sinful of non-believers to the least sinful of believers, and from those of any color to those in any state of mind.

God's team is the home team. God, who never sleeps on His watch, oversees the game each moment of every day and night. He also calls the plays and controls the game in His own way and in His own time. Players who are genuinely interested in improving their daily performances always seek to understand and increase their knowledge of God's Word (the Bible), and yearn to grow closer to Him through His Word. They condition their spiritual muscles by uniting with the official body of God, that being the universal Church established by Jesus Christ to promote and increase the kingdom of God on earth.[12] Consistency in these practices separates the home team from the opposing team.

The separation of players presents two obvious tendencies in our performance. Regardless of the calls made by God, everybody does not play the game in the same way. Neither does everybody play according to all of His calls. These two factors have always separated the home team from the opposing team and contributed to their operation in the game as two major leagues: the heaven-bound league of Jesus and the hell-bound league of Satan. Both leagues constantly recruit players throughout the game.

Though God is gravely concerned about our choice of league commitment at all times, He always responds as an equal opportunity provider to each member of both leagues. Otherwise, some players would have only bright and happy days, while other players would have only dark and gloomy days.

Our spiritual ability to endure the raging storms of life is the kind of evidence that God looks for as solid proof of our league choice. After all, reliance on God is much of what the game is all about. It is a test of our faith in God through Jesus Christ, and the daily application of that faith in our lives as we seek to do God's will.

A previous comment in this section confirmed that all of us are perfect, but only according to God's plan. The extended reality of that truth makes it plain that we aren't, and were never intended to be a flawless creation of God. Hence we can never be perfect as the Father who bore us.[13] Perfection for us is also impossible because unlike God, our existence is bound by urges and restraints of our human nature. In that sense, all players, from the best of us to the worst of us, are created equal. We are all sinners in the sight of God.

Since our energy is mixed with human power, every now and then we switch our league allegiance. Oftentimes, for lack of commitment to either league, we straddle our allegiance by transferring to a neutral league of players who stand for nothing and fall for anything.

Many of the most active teams in the game, such as those listed, may also be recognized by other names.

Heaven-Bound League Teams	Neutral League Teams	Hell-Bound League Teams
Truth	Evasion	Falsehood
Justice	Silence	Injustice
Faith	Doubt	Disbelief
Love	Isolation	Hate
Compassion	Indifference	Conceit
Good	Pretense	Evil
Hope	Denial	Despair
Peace	Cowardice	War
Unity	Confusion	Division
Obedience	Irresponsibility	Disobedience

Team participation in the game is outstanding among all three of the leagues. Though neither league has a pure membership of full-time committed players, each league does have a mark of distinction that's more stable than the team memberships. Heaven-bound players attempt to walk in the light with God, while hell-bound players run boldly or sneak around with the devil in darkness. Neutral players don't have the guts to walk or run at all; they just crawl to and fro at a shameful rate. Some slither into oblivion.

Personal and group violations are common occurrences in the game of life. Besides those that are totally malicious acts, some violations are deliberate, but not malicious. They are situational, and happen when we are seized by the moment. Quite often we feel compelled to be either complimentary fibbers, who commend poor performances, or sympathetic fibbers, who conceal painful truths from loved ones. Violations of this sort probably amuse God more than doing anything else.

Aside from situational violations, sometimes we just become so tired, weak, worn, and thoughtless that we commit personal and group fouls without awareness. These are unintentional fouls that also happen when we are overly eager or desperate in making our moves. At times, even the best of our intentions result in a misplay, such as doing or saying something that's totally inappropriate when we are abruptly frustrated or offended. Then, too, there are other innocent occasions when we actually think that our actions are appropriate, but they prove to be just the opposite. A classic example is staging a surprise for somebody, only to end up being the one surprised or embarrassed.

Situations of unintentional fouls also include circumstances that force us to foul as a means of survival. The growing intensity of brutal activity may cause God to eventually overlook bodily harm that's inflicted on hard-hearted criminals, but no time soon.

With respect to our ultimate goal, God knows the intent of our hearts and minds long before we foul. As long as we are mentally alert in the game, and because of God's design of human existence, we have an opportunity to clean up our act by forgiving and repenting. At times, however, apologies are not always sufficient for settling our misdeeds.

Players are often benched regardless of any clean-up efforts, or the lack thereof. Worse than the penalty of being benched, some players are also suspended during the game. In either case, the same consolation is ever-present. With or without our petititions, God continues His generosity by giving us a thousand more chances to remain or to become champions of His cause. Once we use each thousand of our chances in additional fouls, He always gives us a thousand more.

All players alternate between being benched, suspended, or on probation during the entire game. Whereas all players do not sin at the same level, at no time is the playing status based on team allegiance. If the foul fits, home team players are banned from public participation just as easily as members of the opposition, and opposing team members play on probation just as easily as members of the home team. The main point is our penalties never isolate us from God. Every player has equal and permanent access to God through Jesus Christ.

The moral and immoral majority of game participants play on probationary status because they are allowed to escape direct penalties more often than other players. Many thank God for their escape; others claim their unscathed deliverance from ill-fated situations as a stroke of luck. Whether fouls are known publicly or not, God is always aware of our actions. More often than not, especially when we think that we are sliding by on luck or some rabbit's foot, God is probably allowing time for our conscience to work.

Most penalized players return quickly to their positions on the public stage of God's turf. Unfortunately, a great number of players foul to the point of losing their privilege of public participation. Some are grounded off-stage for life. In both instances, these players also have the advantage of either joining, remaining, or renewing their membership with the home team. Even convicts, while grounded on death row, have converted to the home team.

Eventually, all players are retired from the game as a finality of life on earth. Retirement results in players receiving the ultimate penalty or the ultimate reward. The difference is a matter of whether we transcend in our earthly departure to a lower destination or a higher destination.

The distance that we fall is never too far from God. The number and consequences of fouls are less important than reasons that cause players to foul in the first place. Fouls that are maliciously intended happen because of two voids in our lives. The first is our focus on God and the teachings of the Master, Jesus Christ. This void causes our game performance to be similar to that of an outfielder in a baseball game who, in taking his eyes off the ball, misjudges the catching distance. We often misjudge our sinning distance from the opposition and fall flat on our faces because, in the process, we lose sight of God. Yet, whether we ask for help or not, God is always in the midst of our situations. He is also the reason that we are able to stand again.

12

The second void is a matter of spiritual protection and preservation. Thus, the game of life becomes more distinguished as a game of glamour with pre-established dress codes.

All players are instructed to wear the full armor of God.[14] Though dressing up for God is one of our better efforts in the game, we are forever haunted by a common problem. The historical character of man has always proven that our human flesh is too weak to bear the full weight of God's uniform. This weakness leaves one option that merits our full consideration. We should always stretch our spiritual selves toward making an honest effort to please God. This means that we should try to keep on a few of the uniform pieces that we do manage to wear, rather than shed them bit by bit for our temporary comfort and pleasures. There can be no doubt that the longer we try to wear some of His armor, the happier God is with us.

Unlike the home team uniform, the outfit of the opposition is made from a lightweight fabric that changes colors very easily. In fact, the devil's uniform is a "wash and wear" homemade suit that enables his players to change their images several times a day. In contrast to the virtues of faith, hope, love, and others that adorn the armor of God, the uniform of Satan is patched with the many forces of evil. The more comfortable and persistent that players become in wearing this uniform, the more God probably grieves.

Aside from having team uniforms, both teams are also supported by their own cheerleaders and fan clubs. In the midst of their efforts to attract, distract, and convert other players, God waits patiently for opposing team players to declare themselves as free agents and commit to the home team. Satan's hopes are quite the contrary.

The acquisition of new converts does not necessarily increase the membership of either team. Occasionally, the additional intake of new converts is no more than an even exchange of players. The same is also true in cases of returning veterans. Trade-offs of players happen frequently because the headquarters and branches of each team have revolving doors through which players come and go at will. When team players switch their allegiance back and forth on a steady basis, they more or less stabilize the tradition of balance between the two memberships. The down side of this situation is the tendency of some church congregations to ignore gradual departures from their memberships.

Overall, much of what God desires is for our personal and spiritual appearance to be of such nature that we are easily recognized as His children. Despite our low visibility in several areas that are crucial to winning the game, one certainty remains. If our faith matches the smallest grain of a mustard seed, the ultimate reward of eternal life is always within our reach.[15] Furthermore, whenever we suit up with any amount of faith, we can perform bravely in the game because home team players are not endowed with fear.[16]

In the final analysis, God engineers our lives until we finish the course of His purpose. Some courses are longer than others because some of His purposes require more time than others to complete. On that basis, God determines the length of our course to the exact amount of time that He allows us to play the game. Methuselah had 969 years, while Jesus had barely thirty-three years. The difference in the quality between those two life spans confirms a social truth. It is not how long we live that counts; it's what we do while we live.

The Apostle Paul emphasized love as the greatest of

all virtues.[17] Since Jesus is a sacrificial gift of love given to the world directly by and of God, our purpose in the game of life is best served with love. There is no greater passion to sustain our faith in God through Jesus Christ.

The Best of Four Quarters
(Social Foundations of the Game)

High school class reunions breed memories of old times with the fanfare of a stroll down memory lane. The journey is a sentimental route to a cherished past of hairdos and fashions that are no longer stylish, and of the neighborhood grocery store that no longer exists. Almost from the start, laughter erupts among old classmates and becomes as contagious as winter colds. Ever so often, recall of infamous pranks is mixed with remembrance of long ago friends whose whereabouts remain unknown. At other times, before the jubilant mood swings all the way back to the "here and now" of those who are gathered, somebody is bound to say, "Those were the good old days!"

How soothing it is, indeed, when the good old days return us to the sentimental smells, sounds, and ways of much earlier times, especially those of our childhood. Childhood is the basic era of life. Yet, whether we were poor or rich, the good old days that we reap from our childhood aren't about poverty or wealth. For those of us whose childhood was laden with illness or other misfortunes, the good old days are hardly about surviving hardships.

In the broadest sense of life, the good old days aren't really about the quality of childhood at all. They are simply memories that provide customary breaks from a present time of life.

16

Time begets change, and change begets different lifetimes such as the lifetime that separates prehistoric man from modern man. Different lifetimes also occur within our personal life-spans. As time creeps more and more into the gap between our present and past, the better portions of our past eventually become the good old days. They become the thrilling moments of an unforgettable time that separates one period in our lives from another.

The average course of one's life can be divided from several perspectives. According to the ancient "Riddle of the Sphinx," we transcend three stages: morning, when man walks on four legs as a baby; afternoon, when man walks on two legs as an adult; and evening, when man walks on three legs in old age with a cane.

Stages of human life are also compared with seasons of the earth; spring and summer are symbolic of the beginning and fullness of life, and fall and winter are symbolic of the decline and finality of life. There are also biophysical seasons or periods of life that control our maturation and childbearing years.

In the game of life, the projected average life span of eighty years is broken into four periods of playing time. Each period is a quarter of twenty years. Players who endure the fourth quarter accumulate a fortune of good old days from three previous quarters, and one more if God extends their purpose into overtime.

Curiosity is the forerunner of exploration. The first cry of newborn babies is the magnificent sound that begins the first play period of the game. Crying is also the official language of all babies, that is until they begin to smile and stare. Along with staring themselves into familiarity with their immediate surroundings, babies develop a greater urge. They are compelled by the power of curiosity to touch, rip apart, and pull on everything that is within their reach.

Those activities and others are preludes to a higher level of the human purpose. Close to ten months later, babies begin their lifetime expedition with a smile and the first of their independent steps.

Before ending their first ten years on God's turf, babies are already children who dress themselves, make their beds, eat with silverware, and cross the street alone. They still cry and smile, but they do more than stare to question their surroundings. Speaking in the actual language of their native land, they ask neverending questions to satisfy their curiosity.

Since children are born in the arena with an automatic inside scoop on who's who in the game, their curiosity tackles the "whats, whens, whys, and hows" of life.

Prior to leaving childhood years behind, children score quite a bit as players in the game. They learn many of the dos and don'ts of life, and have a great number of first-time experiences. They also begin to accumulate the first of those good old days to which they will return in thought, again and again.

The second half of the first quarter has an added agenda of all the teenage years. Curiosity embraces a new level of peer involvement, and even helps in defining personal and social values at this point in the game. Different exposures of young players to various climates of the home, school, church, and broader community help to cultivate these players' ability to make significant choices. The extent to which curiosity dominates the new freedom of teenagers to make choices is crucial to how they play the remaining quarters in the game. In the meantime, the number of their good old days continues to rise.

By no means, however, is curiosity a one-quarter factor in the game. It is a basic instinct that stimulates players to explore life more, quarter after quarter.

Most traits, when developed in the first quarter, create a supportive connection for players between their play periods. They cause players to be consistent in their behavior from one quarter to the next. This idea suggests, as an example, that players who demonstrate independence during childhood are likely to show a sense of independence for the duration of the game. Habitual behavior is partially responsible for creating the character by which players are known.

Regardless of how stable a player's character is from one play period to another, each quarter contributes its own measure of personal, social, moral, and spiritual influence.

Though curiosity is an opening feature of the game, there are other major attractions in the first quarter of play that are just as important. Besides producing the woven fabric from which all players come, the first quarter bears the chisel of life that shapes the beginning of whoever and whatever all players become. It also introduces the original blueprint for laying the solid foundation that every player needs to help their success in the game. Ideally, this foundation begins with parental love, guidance, and discipline.

Without doubt, parents have a huge presence in the game of life. However, the social distance between parenting trends of today and those of yesteryear has been magnified by the miles of time, thus presenting another model of the good old days.

Once upon God's civilized turf, parenting had a stronger base of command. Children seemed to have had a higher regard for parents as authority figures. They also showed a greater understanding of parental roles and responsibilities. For the most part, respecting any adult was a way of life for children. This was especially true when being disciplined by adults other than their parents.

At a much earlier time, parenting was effective because parents were parents and children were children: parents controlled and remained in control, and children either obeyed or accepted the consequence of their disobedience without much resistance; parents were heard, and children were seen; parents taught by example, and children learned appropriate behaviors; parents asked the questions, and children responded in a cautious and gentle way (whether truthful or not); parents rode in the driver's seat, and children didn't have cars; parents said "no," and children said nothing; parents said jump, and children knew how high; parents were adults, and children were not.

Within the last fifty years, those images of parent-child relationships definitely shifted on American soil. Social grounds of good and sufficient cause may include society's shift from pure cotton to polyester wool; on the other hand, maybe not. Despite any possibility of such an absurdity, one point is obvious. At some time amid other social change, parenting gradually merged with a newness that invaded the American way of life.

Old-fashioned parenting held its fame until the late 1950s. By the sixties, parenting had already been slightly contaminated by the popularized "generation gap." At that time, the effect was no more than a pseudo-communication problem between parents and their children. Yet children were generally allowed to develop a false sense of independence, while parents became lax in raising children up in the way that they should go. Some parents, in a more recent determination to raise their children "differently," have ended up with children whom they actually fear.

In addition to the generation gap, many other factors emerged that impacted the parenting process. This series of factors began with Chief Justice Earl Warren delivering the opinion of the United States Supreme Court in the 1954 school desegregation case of *Brown v. Board of Education of Topeka*. Shortly thereafter, Elvis Presley rocked the nation with a pair of blue suede shoes, and the presidential assassination of John F. Kennedy shocked the entire world. Between the last two events, Dr. Martin Luther King, Jr. was directing a massive movement that later redefined our American values. Ultimately, the reign of hippies and Afro-hairdos ushered us into a brand new day of parenting. The impact is still visible.

Effectiveness of modern-day parenting trends becomes more of an issue when attention is given to other realities of the parenting process itself. The village concept, once practiced as the neighborhood standard for raising children, almost diminished with black and white television. The stern look from mother to child that was once a direct command to "stop now or die" is practically a misdemeanor, but whipping children is definitely an outright felony.

High incidence of alcohol, child, and drug abuse among family members, haste and impatience, parental anxiety and other personality disorders, and even rush hour traffic have also had a tremendous impact on the parenting process. All too often, as compensation for those factors, offerings of material gifts replace parental love, guidance, discipline, and other responsibilities on the home front. Meanwhile, teacher apathy, resignation, and termination replace student discipline in the school setting.

In a large segment of society, traditional boundaries of freedom and control that were once enforced to keep children in their place have been changed to accommodate the imposition of new social trends and legal restraints. Consequently, the current generation of children grows up with greater freedoms of self-expression, ownership, and personal involvements. As the "3-T" generation, children have their own television, telephone, and toilet.

Perhaps the impact of video games, movies, and televised programs on parenting is the most ignored. The total effect of these attractions continues to influence a higher level of disrespect between parents and children. In isolated cases, the results have been drastic. After partying together from dusk to dawn, a few parents and children kill each other off.

Except for differences in age and size, there's very little that separates parents from their children. They frequently display the same level of authority in making decisions, unless the matter involves who brings the bacon home. However, in desperate times of seeking instant gratification that requires parental approval, children have no problem with being children. They even cry, pout, and have temper tantrums; some run away from home.

When viewing the total picture of parenting against its modern background, the parental process becomes a more positive aspect of the game because of a coexisting population that stands as an exception. In that population, parents are parents and children are children; the difference is visible to the naked eye. That difference also causes fewer children to land in our judicial system as juvenile delinquents.

The far-reaching effects of parenting in the game can never be overestimated. Parenting will always have an impact on how children play the game, especially in the quarters of their adulthood. As a tool of social change, parenting will always impact the attitudes and behaviors of society and its future players.

Primary in the total run of all parental effects is the level of attention that's given to promoting and securing a relationship with God. Any effort of this sort requires commitment to the standard set forth by the "Parent" of all parents; "Train up a child in the way he should go: and when he is old, he will not depart from it."[18]

Though rising to the challenge of raising children will hardly be achieved with total perfection, consistent opposition to the aforementioned rule weakens parenting to being just another ideal of the game that's largely ignored, even if by only one parent.

Exploring the possibilities of life is a grand adventure. The experience of learning to ride a bicycle is an adventure in fun that can also become an extremely difficult and dangerous situation. As a means of being protective, some parents teach their children to ride with the aid of training wheels. In other cases, parents are actually the safeguards. They hold onto the bicycle to steady the child and the bike until the child is able to master the two-wheel ride alone.

From a side glance, the experience of mastering the two-wheel ride on a bicycle is somewhat similar to mastering the game of life. Both experiences normally begin in the first quarter, but several sets of training wheels are used in learning the game of life. Instead of being store-bought, the training wheels for mastering life are manufactured directly through exposure to home and school environments and the world-at-large. The greater similarity is that parents and all other adults are expected to ensure the safety of children.

The main difference between the two learning experiences is in the ride itself. After the first quarter, mastering a two-wheel ride and life is more similar to mastering a horseback ride, simply because a horse is larger.

Falling is a common error in life. Whether from a bicycle or horse, the experience of falling without any forewarning is always a possibility that may or may not relate directly to how well the ride is mastered. Regardless of the cause, getting up requires one effort and continuing the ride requires another.

Riding the continuous wave of life has about the same consequences, but involves much more personal and group activity. Besides falling, our errors in life include a lot of fumbling and stumbling. Based on our circumstances, getting up or steadying ourselves and moving on with our responsibilities and goals require certain adjustments. Determining those adjustments and knowing how and when to make them are necessary steps for recovery.

Equipping young players with the basics of life completes the total task of the home, school, and church for the first quarter. Though the ability of young players to manage life is quite premature at this stage of the game, the first real test of mastery always begins during the high school years.

At some time, all first-quarter players are faced with a need to declare their post-high school intentions. This task poses a dilemma for many players because of conflicting interests and other factors. One of the other factors is many of these players don't have a clue when it comes to deciding their future. The situation is more complicated for high school dropouts because most are lacking in skills and ambition.

Whether first-quarter players decide their future

freely, under parental pressure, or not at all, the first twenty-year period of life ends the first quarter of the game.

Once the second quarter begins, players enter the major league of life. The comfort zone of home converts into a new field of responsibilities, needs, and pursuits. Ready or not, the basic set of training wheels are removed for good. Though parents remain supportive, they are no longer held accountable for being safeguards. For the first time in the game, players are officially on their own and free to explore their options in life as adults.

Neither childhood nor adulthood minimizes the fact that each quarter is played on a field of disadvantages as well as advantages. Upon beginning the second quarter, many players are still taunted by the handicap of being too young for some experiences and, at the same time, too old for others. This nagging dilemma, though brief and more common for teenagers, is a major upset for players who have longed for adulthood since their thirteenth birthday.

At the age of twenty-one, those players invariably expect and demand that their adulthood be recognized with total respect. Anything less may cause some of them to develop abnormal feelings of rejection, frustration, and insecurity. Attempts to conceal or compensate for those feelings include periods of bitterness, isolation, and making choices that may have damaging consequences.

In response to young people who show maturity or immaturity in their pursuits, senior players often share the sentiment that youths have their whole life ahead of them. Even as a message of optimism, the reality of that view has a standard time limit.

The second quarter is practically the last opportunity in the game for players to comfortably enjoy and rely on the advantage of having time on their side. Accordingly, it is the best quarter for planning life-long dreams. Beyond the planning emphasis, however, the grandest event of this game period always occurs with the birth of brand new players.

The second quarter is also a very different time in the game. Players are practically forced to meet the world head-on for its total worth. Somewhere in the course of exploring various aspects of life, they learn that living in the real world is more than riding to the prom in a chauffeured limousine. From the magnitude of this "polite" awakening, these players develop a greater sense of social tradition and become more responsive to learning and following the rules of social order. Meanwhile, another primary lesson of this quarter is learning the value of planning for a "rainy day."

As unpredictable as rainy days may be, they are never an option in life. They are a natural craft of God that come with His promise to supply all of our needs.[19] Yet, within the realm of human experience, we speak of rainy days as potential times of woe. True to the natural course of life, sometimes the rains of woe catch us completely off our guard. Nevertheless, any rainy day is a part of God's plan and purpose. The fact that He allows us to contribute freely to the cause of some of our social and personal woes adds another point about the population of second-quarter players.

All players, having gone through some basic preparations for life, are expected to develop a sense of moral conscience. School children have enough experiences during the game to learn, understand, and know, for instance, that cheating on a classroom test is wrong. Otherwise, a few of them who do not cheat probably would, and some who do cheat would probably not waste their time and energies on concealing their efforts. Neither would they feel the need to respond so quickly with untruths upon being caught or implicated in the act.

The worst response when caught in deliberate acts of wrongdoing is showing regret for having been caught without any concern or remorse for having done something wrong. This tendency in children helps to create a climate for potential problems in the second quarter. The probability is higher that some players who constantly cheat and lie as children will cheat and lie eventually with criminal intent. The woes of life, however, are not always related specifically to pre-existing patterns of behavior.

Our rainy days and falls in life share the same profile of cause and effect. The challenge of each event interferes with our comfort and joy. For obvious reasons, these events are never the best of times; and, even more frustrating, they do not occur on any particular schedule. As a result, facing challenges in early adulthood can be a difficult task because many of the players are handicapped more by inexperience than by age. Other than being frustrated by the challenges of life, there is the frustration of planning for life. Early attempts by young adults to establish their lifetime comfort zone may prove to be difficult because of general deficiencies such as the inability to make wise decisions.

In any event, difficult situations require a great deal of effort, and adults are not always committed to going an extra mile. More often than not, the current generation of young adults will not hesitate to give up on a situation, regardless of gains or losses. Instead of seeking resolution, they evade significant issues and resort to impulsive actions that magnify their problems. Insufficient effort, if not acting in haste, causes the thrill of being newlyweds to turn into the pain of divorce.

If players are unable to deal appropriately with rainy days and falls that are self-made, then there is little hope that they will do better under circumstances over which they have no control. When the excitement of landing a job for the first time becomes the agony of unemployment because of a lay-off, twittling thumbs may be the basic response. If, however, this is the only response, then a home eviction notice will probably not be far behind.

Life is filled with routines and potentials that have positive and negative consequences. In the same sense, scattered showers of calm and turbulence are destined events of life that occur with or without a forecast. Within minutes, the joy that comes with winning a million-dollar lottery can be shattered by an evil deed of man or by an act of nature; life goes on according to God's plan.

By way of Biblical orientation, God is the super power of human existence and the force of nature. Hence, everything that happens in life validates God's purpose in man and His presence in the human experience through nature. Inasmuch as God commands the wind and sea, it is only natural to believe that He controls everything.[20]

As a part of God's command, rain serves a distinct purpose in our lives. It activates our line of faith in God and the level of our self-confidence. Hoping and praying to God for rain is what we do best in times of drought. Yet, at the same time, we trod the path of life with confidence because we know that rain stops eventually for everybody's parade.

We also know, as a matter of circumstance, that rain can be just as upsetting as it is uplifting. Any negative outcome from a major downpour of woe is sufficient cause for some of us to lose our confidence. Some of us also tend to lose all sense of happiness and faith.

As a rule of the game, whenever we choose to lose our faith in God, we also resign from our purpose in life. In order to keep up our hope for winning the game, we should be grateful with each ray of sunshine for any degree of survival. This notion brings into focus the final points of coverage on the second quarter.

From any unspecified times in the first quarter through our final moments on earth, we play the game according to our strengths and weaknesses, accomplishments and failures, attitudes, maturity, and values. Despite our level of existence, these factors can enhance or do harm to our image and performance as managers of the human experience.

The task of learning how to manage life effectively is crucial activity of the second quarter because it impacts our ability to win the game. A preliminary step, then, is for players to commit to their roles as adults. The urgency of this effort is noted in Paul's message to the Corinthians: "When I was a child, I spake as a child, I understood as a child, I thought as a child: but when I became a man, I put away childish things."[21]

By design of the game, the second quarter refines our purpose in life and kindles anew our perspectives on life. In addition to being a time for exploring various aspects of life, the second quarter is a time for players to settle themselves into the labor force. Furthermore, it is the time for players to show a sense of self-worth that influences the lives of others in a positive manner. Players would also be wise to direct some attention toward their future years of retirement, health benefits, and other interests related to making their lives worthwhile as senior citizens.

Essentially, life is God's designated teacher for the second quarter. From this particular perspective and any other, life presents different situations in different ways without any guarantee of what the future will bring. Since the challenge of surviving in a world of uncertainty is ever present, we should proceed with caution on a daily basis. Strategies for achieving success in this effort include the following recommendation from the players' manual: "Lay not for yourselves treasures upon earth. . . . But lay up for yourselves treasures in heaven. . . . For where your treasure is, there will your heart be also."[22]

The aforementioned recommendation reinforces God's exact order that we have no other God before Him. This reinforcement is urgent for all players, especially those who are bent on profiting by unethical and illegal means. The lesson to be learned is quite simple: we profit nothing when we choose to give up our souls in exchange for worldly gains.[23] Whenever we proceed with this choice, we automatically become weak and ineffective players. We fail to realize that forsaking God in our hearts and minds is a spiritual crime that does not pay because anything to the contrary of God's Word does not work. Regardless of motives, ineffective players who constantly risk losing their souls automatically rank high among the most likely of all players to lose the game.

First impressions are not final. Due to our individual differences and other factors, all of us are not destined to learn the same lessons from life. Neither are we required to learn any lesson at the same time or at the same rate of speed. But we do become burdens in society when the arrogance of a know-it-all attitude prevents us from learning at all. While laziness has the same effect, a tragic deed of ignorance is failing to seek and accept assistance in a time of need. Capable players who are unable to manage life effectively because of willful ignorance create needless problems for themselves and others.

As a process of trial and error, learning involves mistakes. Thus, all players make mistakes along the way. The second quarter just happens to be the customary time when the most common mistakes in life are made most often during the game. Regardless of whenever, wherever, or however often we say and do the wrong thing, we are ultimately accountable for making the world a better place. The most ideal goal, until the last player departs from earth, would be to restore the Garden of Eden to its original state.

Our consequences in life are not always products of our learning efforts or mastery of skills. From time to time, our opportunities are improved or limited by the way that we open and close the umbrellas of life. Whether or not it's a sunshiny or rainy day at the time is of little concern. The same applies to whether or not we act by choice or because of imposing circumstances. The main point is that we stand to succeed or fail according to our attitudes, verbal responses, and other gestures.

Even when we are still, our mannerisms are in motion. They constantly create the portrait from which we are perceived by others. This makes it worthwhile to remember that the manner of our responsive behavior indicates more about our character than our learning efforts ever could. Some of us dare pretend not to care about the consequences of our actions. While we deny feelings of regret, human nature makes it doubtful that we really do not care about how our actions affect or are regarded by others. The record of interpersonal relationships proves that what other people think can make or break our public image. On this basis, insensitivity is a known killer of character.

We often hear that a first impression is a lasting impression. This notion bears an element of truth, but first impressions may not always reflect the genuine nature of a person's character. Sometimes first impressions are intended only as a strategy, such as one planned to begin a courtship. First impressions are also leftovers from emotional displays that lack mature purpose altogether, as the case is so often in verbal attacks. The overall logic is that much of what we experience in life is related to how we approach various situations. This same logic is a seed of thought that defines life as a game.

Life shares the basic format of several sports, one of which is bowling. Given this viewpoint, the final segment of the second quarter features bowling as a base of comparison to further examine the importance of our approach in he game of life. This presentation begins with descriptive information on both games.

Procedural Aspects of Bowling

Albeit a rare occasion, league bowlers who roll a perfect game become national statistics and their photographs become mounted fixtures in their "League house" (bowling center). The thrill of bowling a perfect game is the illusive and yet passionate dream among avid bowlers. The dream is etched so deeply on their hearts and minds that the excitement shows whenever they "suit up" to practice and for league or tournament bowling. For the few who bowl a perfect game, the dream lingers until the next time, even if the next time never happens.

Bowling is an individual and group sport. Each game consists of ten frames. Bowlers have two opportunities per frame (turn) to down a target of ten bowling pins that are positioned about sixty feet from the bowler. Though a perfect game is 300 points, a game of 200 points or better is also a fantastic achievement. A high game of 275 points or better is celebrated about as much as a perfect game because it is almost as rare. League bowlers who down ten pins in each frame of a game also receive official recognition.

Ironically, the first step in bowling is to get into position on the approach. This is the designated area where bowlers pause to focus on everything that they feel will help them to achieve their goal. They often plant their feet in a certain way, focus on their target, secure their fingers/hand/ball position, and establish their overall body pose. Attention is also given to the precise spot for releasing the ball, aim and force of release, hand/arm swing/feet coordination, and surface conditions of the approach. These details and follow-through in releasing the ball contribute to an accurate and smooth delivery of the ball. At least, that is the intention. Most times, the shock of missing the target is not really a total surprise. To a great extent, missing the target is the nature of the game that keeps a bowler's dream alive.

As an organized sport, bowling incorporates several kinds of leagues and tournaments on the basis of age and sex gender. League bowling requires active membership status of anybody who is interested, while most tournament bowling is a qualifying event. All championship and consolation prizes are based on a cut off of high scores achieved by individual or team effort. Every bowler is required to wear bowling shoes, use standard bowling equipment, show lane courtesy to bowlers on the next lane by not stepping out on the approach to bowl at the same time, and comply with all other related guidelines. Failure to do so may lead to disqualification.

Procedural Aspects of the Game of Life

Except in cases of extraordinary circumstances, most eulogistic remarks favor beliefs that place the deceased in heaven. The high frequency of these remarks suggests that heaven must be an unimaginable, big place beyond the skies where families, friends, strangers, and pet animals gather after death. From all that is known and speculated, the distance is so far away that it remains unmeasured from earth.

Heaven's enrollment roster has never been revealed to human eyes, nor has a slate of daily candidates ever been published. Regardless of who has gone there or may be the next in line to go, more players than not probably dream of going to heaven rather than the alternative of being routed to Satan's flaming abode. All heaven-bound hopefuls believe that there is no better finality to death than spending eternity around the throne of God. This belief is more than enough to validate an invitational call to heaven as the ultimate championship prize for any and all believers.

The belief that going to heaven is an accomplishment of unspeakable joy keeps the dream of winning alive for almost any player, but preparing for the journey is not always easy. Our agendas cause a steady flow of environmental and personal static. At times, the interference is so great that prayers to God on our behalf by our parents and others are no more than murmurs, though distinctly heard by God. Louder and clearer prayers of support are all the same because the final determination on who wears the championship crown of eternal life is not based on group effort or support. While praying is a fundamental requirement for all players, the impact of prayer on winning the game of life is a personal matter between God and man.

God's busy schedule includes a day in His courtroom when every player will stand alone in judgment and on his or her own merit.[24] In the absence of an attorney, players must show proof of their individual efforts. That proof represents the degree of light that shines in our works.[25] Thus, a ball is to bowling as our light is to the game of life. Since there is never a substitute judge in God's court of law, only God is in a position to determine whether or not the evidence of all things done by players is sufficient for winning the game. Imperfection is permissible because we are not perfect creatures; we are flesh and bones from head to toe.

Until the actual time of our earthly departure, the game of life is always an individual sport that involves direct and indirect group activity. God controls each person's game and makes it known that all players on His team must first commit their lives to Him through Jesus Christ. The timing is critical because God is the only one who knows exactly how long each player will live. Players who take this all important step early in life may have an advantage of more time for making adjustments, reconciling differences, and settling personal violations.

A main advantage of our commitment to Jesus is its value as a comprehensive game insurance policy. Already paid in full with His blood, this policy is a lifetime guarantee of incredible benefits. It covers all earthly damage that we experience because of our actions and any other force. There is a hitch, however. Unlike policies requiring annual renewal, our responsibility is to renew God's coverage on a daily basis by the seconds of every minute.

The terms of God's insurance plan promote earth as a temporary dwelling place where we get into position and attempt to make the cut for heaven. Thus, we have the full range of earth as a designated approach area where our thoughts, words, and deeds reflect our commitment to the game. Moreover, the lot of our daily performance helps or hinders our suitability for heaven.

As unworthy as we all are to enter the gates of heaven, players make the cut by conditions of God's discretion in awarding the victory of death. Whether our final destination is heaven or hell, there is a chance of experiencing an "after-death" shock. Some players are probably just as surprised by their final landing place as they are by the final destination of others.

So, dream as we may about going to heaven, it's all for naught unless we honestly intend to minimize our violations and tendency of repeating mistakes. Whereas this task is difficult for most of us as players of habit, minimizing our sins may be the one act that we can possibly perfect with practice.

Common Denominators of Both Games

Bowling provides limited proof that "practice makes perfect"; and this adage is totally impractical and "athletically incorrect" in the game of life. Yet, the odds against achieving perfection in either game does not lessen motivation among players who are sincere and passionate about their goals and commitments. They continue to practice and cling to the hope of winning or being as close to perfection as their individual nature allows.

The approach has a dual meaning in both games. It is an area where players get into position and make adjustments or the quality of their efforts. In either case, and under any circumstance, the sloppier players are in approaching a situation, the sloppier the outcome. By the same token, whenever players put their best foot forward in approaching various tasks, the outcome is usually favorable to the situation at hand.

A positive approach, when executed as a genuine effort of good will, trumps a negative approach most times in life. Such an effort makes us more effective in managing interpersonal relationships at home, school, church, work, and in other social settings. In turn, we gain a purer [godly] sense of self-satisfaction. Results of this same effort in resolving verbal conflicts are emphasized in the Old Testament of our manual; "A soft answer turneth away wrath: but grievous words stir up anger."[26] Even public opinion leans toward a positive attitude as being half the cure in times of illness.

God desires that we show our love for Him with the best of our commitment and service; He wants our "best foot" at all times. Declaring our position in this effort on the public approach of life is basic activity of the second quarter. The quality of our effort in acting on God's purpose and our debt of love to Him is always a personal matter of choice, timing, circumstance, and attitude.

By way of commitment to the Ruler of our purpose, there is no better time than during the second quarter for players to acknowledge who is, indeed, "the boss." In terms of accountability, this acknowledgment deserves our firmness, faithfulness, and maturity. The second quarter is also a prime time to decide whether, in our stead, the rocks should show gratitude and praise for God's abounding goodness to us. On this matter, the Gospel according to Luke has already confirmed that if we do not praise God, the stones surely will.[27]

Halfway through the game is not the half-time of life. Life does not get easier just because we become adults. It may neither prove to be more difficult, but the challenges are different and more in number. In the game of life, adulthood exceeds the routine of juggling responsibilities and schedules between family, work, and other social activities. At the end of the first half of the game, adulthood takes us to the third quarter and through the remainder of the game. These transitions place us at another level on the approach platform. Before proceeding with that presentation, there is a period of time between the two halves of the game that cannot be ignored. It serves the same purpose of the half-time break in organized football.

Fans who watch football games from bleachers or by television do various things during half-time. In addition to taking restroom breaks, stocking up on snacks, and making brief telephone calls, these fans recap the best and worst plays of the first half. After exhausting their hindsight wisdom, these same fans proceed to declare a winner for the half-finished game.

High school, college, and professional football can spark quite a stir among fans when a game is being played by two long-time rival teams. Occasionally, fans are in such an emotional uproar that they become queen and king profiteers. Their wagering foresight skips to the point of generating bets on every game yet to be played in that season and the next. Football players are noticeably absent from all of this commotion, but not by incident. They have a private half-time agenda that differs from that of the fans.

Immediately upon ending the second quarter, football teams race to the locker room to recap and regroup on strategies. They analyze inexcusable mistakes and review plays to weaken the strength of their opponents. Most of all, they reaffirm their goal and commitment as a team, that being to put forth their best effort to win the game. Competitive teams, perhaps down by enough points to qualify winning as a miracle, play until the end. They may play tired, but they never forsake their goal of winning.

Half-time in the game of life has a different twist of events. According to the format of this game, all second-quarter players end the first half at the age of forty. The very thought of approaching half a century in age should be enough during the break to add new perspectives on life and refine the old. Players who are sill uncommitted to earning the victory of eternal life have sufficient cause to make this matter a top priority for consideration. At the same time, God's home team players would waste precious time recapping their errors if, all along, there has been follow-through on forgiving and repenting. These two steps assure us that God wipes our slates clean of previous misdeeds. Therefore, we just need to make a half-time game choice about our goal and commitment. **To continue or not to continue: that is the decision to be made.**

Aside from serious aspects of the half-time break, there is the major attraction of a half-time show. A football game is not a game without this feature. Some fans are known to attend a game just for the half-time show. During this event, marching bands strut their stuff and popular entertainers perform. This course of attractions may not be as elaborate in our private lives, but the celebrations can be just as exciting with festive birthday parties.

The game of life has a provision of half-time attractions as well, but not on the same order of marching bands and parties. As an effort to not be completely outdone by tradition, the following presentations were created for our personal half-time attention.

"Thinkin' on the Turf"
(Complimentary Thoughts of the Author)

All calls to God are local, even when they are made from a long distance.

Until we bathe in the richness of God, we are as filthy as He is rich.

Tomorrow never comes and today never goes; what a long wait for yesterday to happen.

If you are where you have never gone, then you aren't there.

Trying to find God is a lost cause because He is not lost; He is always where we place Him in our hearts and minds.

All ye of little faith: Jesus is truly the Son of God, for who else could live and cause such a stir for two thousand years?

Whosoever pursues the cause of God satisfies the cause of human purpose; and whosoever lives the purposes of God preserves his soul throughout eternity.

We cannot live a perfect life; our purpose is but to try.

Man's knowledge of God is no greater than what he believes about God.

God comes to us in many ways and asks that we come to Him in one, that being in faith.

God is great and God is good, but He has two problems; I am only one of them.

Man is born an innocent being to choose between good and evil.

Each day that we walk without talking to God is a mile of joy missed in our journey of life.

A deed of sin contaminates our purpose and ignores the glory of God.

"Ifs for Livin' on the Turf" (Complimentary Thoughts of the Author)

If a free dinner-concert featuring two of your most favorite entertainers were held at the same time when all Christians in your neighborhood were to assemble nearby, where would you choose to go and why?

If you were with a group of friends and they began singing "A Mighty Fortress Is Our God," would you recognize the song and know the words of the first stanza?

If you were required to name twelve books of the Bible, two major prophets, and six disciples who were companions of Christ, could you perform this task without error?

If you had the choice to denounce God as creator of man or die at gunpoint, which choice would you probably make?

If you were obligated to list everything that God does for you in the course of a normal day, what would be the numerical range of things on your list?

Select one response: 0–5; 6–18; 19–24; 25–30; More than 30

If you could choose to be any character in the Bible for the remainder of your life, who would be your choice and why?

If you were given the choice to live as long as Methuselah (969 years) and in good health, why would you accept or refuse that choice?

If you could talk with Judas, Pontius Pilate, and Barabbas in person, what would you say to them?

If you had a chance to hand-deliver a gift of your choice to Jesus, what would you give Him and why?

If you had the choice to live permanently in the time of today, yesterday, or tomorrow, which of these actual times would you choose and why?

If you could sell peace, love, and joy, which of these items would be the most expensive and the least expensive and why?

If you were to give a fortune of a million dollars to one person of your choice, who would that person be and why?

If you could revise the Ten Commandments, what would be your changes and why?

If you were forced to either cheat, lie, or steal to save your life, which would you choose to do and why?

From the minute some football games begin, pending who is scheduled to appear on the half-time show, many fans eagerly await the performance of a particular song or band stunt. In response to fan anticipation, guest entertainers usually save their most popular performance for last. When the moment comes, it is nothing short of being a fan's perfect delight.

The hope of achieving similar results accounts for the following poem being the last presentation in this half-time segment. The overall intention is to inspire all players to either begin or to stay the course of commitment to God, our "Coach for life."

"Reminders for Playin' on the Turf" (Complimentary Thoughts of the Author)

God Has Two Eyes and More

God has two eyes and more;
    One stayed on me, the other on you.
'Tis often we straddle His pathway of light,
    Yet never banned from His endless sight.

God has two ears;
   One belongs to me, the other to you,
That He should hear our voices in prayer
   As we hear others and their burdens share.

God has two shoulders;
   One for me, the other for you,
Upon which we lean yet fail to yield
   And opened heart that favors His will.

God has two arms;
   One is mine, the other yours,
That we should ever be cradled in love
   And spread abroad His peace from above.

God has two legs;
   Dare we, by greed, seize both for us?
That we would walk side by side
   Forsaking His presence in our stride?

Nay! God has two kingdoms;
   One is earth, the other heaven.
While yet thriving on His gift of grace,
   We need make earth like His other place.

   The day when all spectators remain quiet and still until the end of a football game will be the day when we sin no more. Yet, for the while that fans do remain, their stay has two halves. This sheer piece of logic points to a truth of human life; the lifetime of every player on earth has two halves. In the game of life, these halves are sometime shorter and sometimes longer than the projected midpoint of forty years. As unfortunate as the case appears with newborn babies, the midpoint of life is only a minute for those whom God retrieves two minutes after their birth.

Perhaps more important than the half-time of life is the matter of premature departures from the game. Droves of fans leave football games early to escape inside and outside traffic or because the score is so far out of reach for the losing team. Some leave before half-time while others leave during the final two-minute warning of the game. Many leave with a smile on their face and many leave in tears, the typical show of emotions that follow championship games.

Failure of players to last until a particular point in the game of life is due to death. There are many times, however, when death on earth is neither physical nor permanent. Some players walk dead on their feet because of emotional and financial depression. Others are dead in life because of hard-core injuries that were personally or socially induced. The overriding cause in non-physical deaths is the need for these players to discover the healing power of God, and to go the distance to obtain this power of life. The sooner the discovery, the sooner the healing process begins.

Time is God's instrument of change. The third quarter is so full of quick activity that it can be hazardous to our health. Instead of Christmas Day coming every twelve years as it does for first-quarter children, it comes every twelve weeks for third-quarter adults. This is one of the few superficial reversals of life. Instead of players rushing time, they are rushed by time. Eventually time goes by so quickly that plucking the first gray hair from our scalp fails to retard the aging process. In just a few weeks, if not days, ten more gray hairs appear on schedule.

These thoughts may exaggerate the speed of time, but they also support a truth that's worded in an old familiar hymn, "Time is filled with swift transition." The effects of that truth just happen to be more visible after half-time. We may be able to camouflage nature; but as a force of God, time will never be detained.

Each half of the game, as well as each quarter, modifies our time by imposing a different pattern of progressive activity. Throughout the first half, this pattern is the constant transition from childhood to adulthood. In addition to being different, the pattern of change is more complicated in the second half. After players discover the traditional rush of the third quarter, they are challenged more so because, at the same time, they are aging.

Veteran players in the third quarter are often victimized by a time that fuses old and new ways of life. The actual time of transition is so brief that it forces instant learning without the benefit of adequate training wheels. The main probability is that, with or without ample assistance, many aging adults need more time than younger players to make adequate adjustments.

Modern invention is another factor of change that merges the old and newness of life. In the process, children have an edge on adults. While children grow up in the "modern" day, adults must be trained to a new way of life. The irony of this trend is always the same. Invention is basically the output of the same quarter of players who fairly much learn principles of operating new home appliances from a younger generation of players. The art of using home computers still runs the course of this irony because of rapid updates in computer models and software.

Younger generation players are the pride and joy of the third quarter and expert contributors to the novelty of third quarter experiences. They are the generation of children and grandchildren in the game who unscrew child-proof caps without any difficulty. They are also skilled in keeping third-quarter adults young at heart, often using fashions and vocabulary as their main props.

Words spoken as standard English usually gain new meanings with every generation of teenagers. According to recent language used by these masterminds, if a dress is described as "bad," this simply means that the dress is fabulous and fits the wearer perfectly. One of the "baddest" expressions of slang is "the bomb," which has nothing to do with weapons of mass destruction. For the sake of information, the bomb is the superlative of anything that's "bad"; the bomb means the best! Thus, by all accounts, God is "THE BOMB!"

Being forever young at heart has great possibilities and is, therefore, a reasonable goal in life. A much weaker and more temporary mission is the intended goal to be forever young in age. Yet, retention of youthfulness is a major preoccupation among third-quarter players. Their determination in this pursuit includes efforts ranging from cosmetic surgery to extramarital affairs.

After so many years in the game of life, especially after the first half, the desire to look good and healthy is only natural. But a persistent need to appear thirty years younger is superficial and lacks maturity when taken to the extreme of compromising trust.

Immediately after the first half of the game, we begin our descent in life. Matters of financial security, health, and aging that some players ignore because of youthful priorities eventually become prominent and demanding. This pattern of change in our lives is sometimes so abrupt and compelling that it can weaken the strongest of players and strengthen the weakest. The challenges are not the same for every player because they originate under different sets of circumstances, even in cases of death. Whereas life-changing situations seem to be more frequent in the third quarter, some of these situations arise earlier and sometimes later than during the third quarter.

Behavioral trends among many third-quarter players in response to challenges along the downward spiral of life include those summarized in the following checklist:

- Adjusting to a quiet household because the children are grown-ups who have moved away from home.
- Assuming a major role in raising grandchildren.
- Trimming the family budget to accommodate three or more unexpected home repairs or major purchases.
- Seeking ways to accommodate health care needs for a spouse, parents, and/or children.
- Beginning a second career, retraining for changes in job responsibilities, or searching for a second job because of new financial burdens.
- Noticing an increase of illnesses and related deaths among coworkers, classmates, family and friends, neighbors, and significant others.
- Becoming a first-time head of household without any experience in managing household business matters such as banking, paying bills, and filing income taxes.
- Becoming increasingly bored with a life that has little chance of getting any better.
- Feeling abandoned by family and friends.
- Waiting to retire with mixed emotions about life

after retirement or staying busy to avoid the frustration of involuntary retirement.
- Trying to cope with on-the-job stress or marital problems that may or may not include recent divorce proceedings.
- Feeling disappointed, unfulfilled, or useless because life is not going according to plan.
- Wanting to turn back the hands of time because adulthood involves too many demanding responsibilities.
- Coping with the death of a dear friend or family member.

The third quarter is a unique time of discovery because of a higher order of responsibilities, change, and challenges. This shift in the game creates a different order of sun rays and rain drops, but it does not break the common thread of positive and negative situations experienced by the players. Situational responses presented in the preceding list lean toward the more negative challenges among third-quarter players. Some of the more satisfying times for these players include the following activities:

- Planning to get remarried or to finally go on a long overdue honeymoon.
- Awaiting a son or daughter's graduation or wedding.
- Awaiting the birth of a first grandchild or great-grandchild.
- Receiving a post-graduate degree or other honors of distinction.
- Planning to establish a private practice or company.

- Landing a significant job offer, promotion, or pay raise.
- Planning and enjoying quality time with family and friends on a regular basis.
- Engaging in a personal exercise/diet routine that promotes a life of good health.
- Advising children on their life goals.
- Making plans to move into a new home or to renovate current home.
- Finalizing plans related to retirement years.

Players who develop an early sense of responsibility, stability, and self-discipline are better prepared to deal with difficulties as life progresses. Even so, human efficiency does not complete the effort needed for managing life with maximum competence. Of all the many factors that generate success in life management, prayer is always extremely important. Beyond being a daily need for effective living, prayer is one of few factors in the game for which there is no substitute.

Prayer is the basic ingredient of life that sustains us through the thick and thin of human experiences. It is an humbling act of submission to the only one who can give us peace when all else fails. The full essence of prayer, even when our motivation is temporary, insincere, and morally offensive, is an acknowledgment of God and the belief that He is able to do all things.

The urgency of prayer as an essential of the game becomes more of an experience in the third quarter. From childhood through young adulthood, players routinely pray in words rather than in thought. Though routine prayer serves a purpose, third quarter experiences and sentimental moments have a way of changing "routine" prayer to an extent that leads us to yet another discovery.

Every quarter should be a time of discovery when it comes to God, but only through prayer do we make the ultimate discovery in life. As an exercise of faith, prayer leads us to discover who God is and what He does in the miracles and tragedies of life. Until we grasp this reality of prayer, our pursuits in life remain as shallow as vain attempts to manipulate the aging process.

In the absence of prayer, God automatically attends to human needs, especially those of children. He makes it possible for them to adjust quickly and comfortably to life-altering challenges. Besides the obvious advantage of being young, these players perform with more resilience than older players in times of physical and emotional tragedies. Although their resilience is not usually a by-product of faith and prayer, it is a product provided to them directly by God.

The capacity to rebound from the dark side of life by faith and prayer is more visible among third-quarters players. This tendency may be due to the average playing time needed in the game for spiritual maturity.

One quarter in the game barely allows enough time for young players to develop in-depth relationships, self-reliance, or faith. These are the historical properties of adulthood that support players through the second half of the game. This area of development is one of the many advantages that third-quarter adults have over younger players. However, the absence of this advantage among young players during traumatic situations reveals the hands of God even more as He softens their recovery.

A toddler who is orphaned certainly senses a loss of parents, but appears to adapt rather quickly to the opened arms of substitute parents. Teenagers who sustain permanent handicaps are less likely than adults to wallow in self-pity. Rather than reconciling initially to a limited lifestyle, teenagers proceed more willingly in rehabilitative efforts. Adults, more so than children, often refuse to pursue their options under such circumstances and, in the meantime, proceed to become bitter human beings for life.

Children, in particular, have a broader and more immediate network of family and community support for assistance and comfort. God made grandparents the leading stars in that network, and they always seem to know exactly what to do in any kind of situation. Thus emerges the fourth quarter and a generation of expert players.

Jesus taught us to pray for a reason. Sixty years of human experience qualifies grandparents and all other peers of the fourth quarter as natural experts on life. Among these experts players, many with proven records of invaluable service are tossed to the curb of social position and clout because of their age. This action, justified or not, takes place despite an existing wealth of knowledge that cannot be dismissed quite as easily.

Due to their lifetime experiences, the fourth-quarter population of grandparents, sports wizards, and the political-minded owns the bulk of worldly wisdom. Their seasoned ability of recall kindles the kind of front porch and barbershop chatter that leads to analyzing past and current conditions of the world and all relevant issues. Many of these players provide accurate details on why particular efforts worked or failed to work through the years. They further dramatize how the world could become a better place.

As the older "been there, done that" generation, fourth-quarter players are a notch higher than being advanced rookies. They are "professional" players, kicking off the Pro Bowl of life with personal records of God's purpose in the game. Their private stash of memories about the good old days and other experiences clarifies the occurrence of all natural and human events as part of a greater plan already foreseen and implemented by God.

While most of these players are successful in adjusting to lingering regrets, a significant number of fourth-quarter players confine themselves to a life dominated by memories of regret. Beyond these situations, many fourth-quarter players reflect on their careers while enjoying the fruit of their labors in retirement. They also help others who depend on benefits provided by somebody else's labors. From this perspective, many players reflect, too, on how they managed to survive the most severe storms of life and helped others through their downpours. They also reflect on their peers yet lost in the floods of life.

Survival in the game of life is not always about overcoming a major obstacle, rather the more simple things in life can become major obstacles. Before the fourth quarter ends, survival for any number of players is a matter of remembering their name.

Among other dramatic changes that take place, self-reliance shifts to greater reliance on God. The overall effect brings into clear view the "by and by" stage of life, theretofore known only from a titled hymn. In response to a newly felt debt of gratitude, many players gravitate to God with renewed fervor. They learn that waiting on the Lord in prayer is a means of gathering renewed strength to complete their journey on earth.[28] Those who would be expert advisors already consider prayer as the core of all spiritual wisdom.

The reality of being in the final play period of life motivates players in different ways. In addition to reminiscing about the past, some players take full advantage of their senior years. Their activities run the gamut of traveling, volunteering time and service to charitable causes, enrolling in adult classes, taking on new hobbies, and affiliating with senior citizen groups.

In a more defining sense, life begins to come full circle for fourth-quarter players. Aging is a constant part of that process and has potential for being a major challenge in this quarter. It reverts a significant number of players to childhood in more ways than one, sometimes in illness and sometimes in physical change. Until modern invention includes body machinery to counteract human aging, senior players are likely to be diapered and toothless prior to leaving the game.

Complications related to aging are a leading cause for final departures among fourth-quarter players, but this situation does not make them the smallest population in the game. This rank goes to the population of players who have advanced beyond their eighty years. Their longevity in life adds two points about the general format of the game. The first to be stated is the more obvious.

Whereas the fourth quarter is the final quarter of the game, it is not the final period of play. The capacity of players to complete the game of life in overtime makes the second point all the more significant.

In organized sports, overtime is an extension of time designated for individual players and teams to break tied scores. The beauty of overtime in the game of life is not just the fact that it happens; it is more a matter of when it happens. Therefore, the all-important point is that overtime does not automatically occur after the fourth quarter.

All participants in the game of life play in overtime throughout the entire game by God's choice. Each close call experienced in life is a reality of overtime. Surviving surgery against the odds or a narrow escape from being killed in an automobile wreck only begins the countless number of overtimes allotted to us in life. The greater truth is that the major portion of overtime is the post-period of play that follows each of our sins.

God has a way of punctuating our purpose with His tactics of preserving life. Therefore, overtime is every second that God allows us to live and every quarter that He allows us to play. Conclusively, overtime is not the post-period of four quarters; it is the best of four quarters.

Movin' from Atozee
(Moral Foundations of the Game)

Life in the big city features all kinds of benefits and pleasures for players in the game of life. Employment and educational opportunities, neon lights and shopping malls, and offerings of various transport services and residential housing are the basics. Provisions of leisure time activities are equally appealing. Players both far and near find excitement in wading through traffic jams just to join the clamor and fun of major league games.

For a few years during my childhood, Atozee existed in my mind as a place of such excitement. It was thought to be a huge city in Georgia because people either cooked, ate, made, owned, or said everything from Atozee. Some even moved everything from Atozee. Until I was about six years old, little did I know that Atozee was a figure of speech used to exaggerate everything in the world from "A to Z." This discovery was one of the biggest disappointments in my life; I had nurtured great visions of one day asking my mom to take me to Atozee.

Growing up brings about a change in how we perceive people, places, and things. In another situation, my tenth grade Latin teacher was one of my idols. I had her signature and her way of talking and walking down pat. I dreamed of owning a 1954 green-and-white Ninety-eight Holiday Oldsmobile as she did, and majoring in Latin upon entering college. I also acquired her passion for drinking Coca-Colas to the extent that I drank an average of six a day.

My other intentions of following in my idol's footsteps were soon forgotten. I initially majored in mathematics, and my first automobile was a 1964 turquoise Bonneville Pontiac. However, even after discovering that she was sipping one Coke on most school days, my addiction to Coca-Cola continued for several years.

Change is a move waiting to happen. Perception is but one human feature that changes with growing up. Our aspirations and level of maturity also change from a point of childhood perspective to a point of adult sensibility. Just as the Apostle Paul, we grow with a greater sense of clarity and understanding.[29]

Growing up and growing old is what happens in life, but adulthood has merit only if learning takes place along the way. As years come and go, we eventually learn from the reality of time that life and the world are in a constant state of motion, and that few things in life remain the same. This discovery further confirms change as a basic element of human experience.

Fewer players in the game of life are in a better position to absorb the full impact of change than fourth-quarter players. Three quarters of social exposure to the world certifies them as historians of social transition. These are the players who have experienced the before and after effects of change, if only by past times of the good old days. Such experience enables the ability to trace the impact of change on society from a positive and negative perspective.

Through their lens of social history, players who are currently in the fourth quarter of the game may agree that American society was on a roll in the 1950s. We had recently cleared the remnants of World War II. Ike was the presidential household name, Motorola TV climbed in household sales, and Stella Dallas was a popular soap opera that captivated household audiences. In the years since, we have thrived on a climate of liberation that has had tremendous consequences, some of which are now seen as unintended. Whether or not some consequences are now regretted is a matter of social conscience.

We often receive more than we plan for in the game of life. At times, the surplus of consequences works against our purpose. The climate of liberation that now characterizes our national spirit is proof. In some instances of our moral conduct, our social tolerance has risen to a level that misinterprets and violates the history of our struggles to be a free people.

Our struggles toward becoming a liberated society began before our birth as a nation with efforts to free ourselves from governance of the British Crown. Since declaring our independence in 1776, a lengthy series of civil protests has been stored in our history. Many of these protests were staged to safeguard our union as a democracy. They included specific attempts to define, assure, and protect fundamental liberties provided to the American citizenry by the United States Constitution.

Some of the most potent moves to correct the imbalance of social standards occurred in the fifties. First among national headlines was the celebrated case of Brown v. Board of Education of Topeka that sought to end racial discrimination in public education. The outcome was a 1954 ruling by the United States Supreme Court that declared the doctrine of "separate but equal" unconstitutional.[30]

The impetus of that ruling changed our democratic behavior in a number of ways, yet not enough to erase our national deficit of social unity and moral conduct. Hardly

58

had national attention been exhausted on the 1955 lynching of Emmett Till before a bold move was made by Mrs. Rosa Parks in Montgomery, Alabama. Mrs. Parks is remembered for her arrest in 1955 after refusing to yield her seat on a local bus to a white man. This incident ignited the Civil Rights movement and a benefit package that promoted democratic ideals. Included were the Civil Rights Acts of 1964 and 1965 that received the presidential endorsement of Lyndon Baines Johnson.

Under the committed leadership of Dr. Martin Luther King, Jr., and scores of other front line defenders during the Civil Rights era of the 1960s, there was a nation-wide campaign to attack all forms of social injustice. Bandwagon effects of that era continue with efforts to protect the rights of women, children, parents, students, teachers, and members of the gay community.

Through struggles stained with blood, sweat, and tears, we did manage to move toward being a more civil people in the domain of human rights. We have also continued to grow in number as a society with benefits of modern technology and medical research. Unfortunately, amidst our moves toward becoming a kinder and gentler nation of modern means, our moral standards began to be slighted by another kind of agenda. We are already a society that is fearful of leaving our cars and homes unlocked. We have a specialized work force that focuses less on work ethics. Consequently, we are an expensive society that pays more and receives less in quality and service.

These and other factors are taking a toll on the entire structure of our social systems. Otherwise, we would not be challenged by issue that divide us as a nation, family, school system, government, or church. As much as we join in the pursuit of life, liberty, and happiness, we remain at odds about how to best achieve that goal.

Terrorism is not the greatest threat in the game of life. In the absence of faith, morals decline; and in the absence of morals, societies decline. This is the story of Sodom and Gomorrah and soon to be the story of American society unless we stand true to our motto: "In God we trust." This is the story of the Israelites who doubted the work of God through Moses and soon to be our story if we shrink further in our faith. This is the story of ancient Rome in its fall from fame as the master empire of the world. This, too, is soon to be our story and that of the modern world if we continue to fail in our primary responsibilities to God. Lest we forget, God has proven that all of these predictions can happen.

Thoughts of the world coming to an end are voiced more in the fourth quarter than in any other quarter of the game. Senior players frequently respond with such ideas when they receive payback for times of declaring their parents, teachers, and all other adults as being outdated. They further complain that the world is "going to the dogs." This particular sentiment reflects an advanced level of the generation-gap that firmly places senior players in the "by and by" era of understanding in the game. Some players never mature to this point.

Every first-quarter population plays throughout the game by its own personal, social, and moral code of ethics. By the time players settle into the fourth quarter, their individual and collective concepts of reality are always precisely different than those of younger generation players. A main side effect of aging in the game is that the society once owned and controlled by senior players changes so fast that most days in the fourth quarter prompt a new way of life.

From a moralistic viewpoint, the game of life is played in a constant state of confusion. The task of separating good from evil, up from down, left from right, apples from oranges, and cotton from wool becomes complicated with time. This hardship is caused by the thoughts and decisions of third-quarter players. In turn, their behaviors become the standards by which we proceed from A to Z as a society. Major complaints regarding the way of life are more commonplace among second and fourth-quarter players. Second-quarter players usually earn the distinction of being the makers or breakers of social harmony.

Perceptions have quite a bit to do with our moves in the game of life. They develop the character of nations and generate national stability and change. Whatever our lot may be, perceptions are forever in the shadows of our progress and relapse.

Various aspects of our move to be a land of opportunity, as in "the land of the free and the home of the brave," continue to work against our purpose. Our perceptions are largely to blame. In all fairness, however, seldom is the time when players can perceive the total scope of a situation and possible consequences. In our course of evolving as a melting pot, we evidently underestimated several realities of accommodating massive diversity, beginning with the abolishment of slavery. Consequently, our struggling days in American society are far from being over.

Unfortunately, in projecting images of the American dream, we have evolved as a materialistic society. Accordingly, our tolerance has drifted to a level where we deliberately engage in compromising our religious and political integrity. The task of reassigning God in the "separation of church and state" becomes increasingly difficult with each attempt. Amid such vain attempts, our native character is being jeopardized by a gradual decline in our moral discipline. We all but glamorize many criminal offenders and exploit episodes of indecent behavior for the sake of public entertainment.

Another effect of our melting pot sensation is the adaptation of our moral conscience to a time when we blend sense and sin without much discretion or hesitation. Supporting evidence is logged from the White House to the courthouse, from presidential misconduct to removal of the Ten Commandments from governmental view, from legalizing abortion to soft-pedaling corporate corruption, and from taking prayer out of public schools to "priestly" molestation of altar boys.

In addition to facing these challenging realities, we are afflicted with a number of unsettled concerns. Three issues in particular have worldwide implications and, therefore, merit review within the confines of our moral character and strength. The first to be presented relates to the impact of our move toward mainstreaming American society.

Total inclusion, as opposed to selective exclusion, is an ideal of the game that has gained significant favor only in recent decades. Thus far, our latest preliminaries of good faith include funding medical treatment, rehabilitation, and training programs for isolated populations of alcoholics, drug addicts, and victims of AIDS.

Regardless of these benevolent and sympathetic attributes, we are still struggling with appropriate perceptions of social inclusion and moral acceptance. Ideally, these two concepts should be the same in principle and practice. Instead, our move to accomplish an all-inclusive society is being downgraded with allowances for immoral behavior. Upon occasions, there is a tendency to confuse immorality with moral tolerance. The gravity of this situation highlights a need for players on the home team and the opposition to stand firm on God's laws with love and mediation.

In response to this need, we can no longer afford to make moral concessions for the sake of popular appeal. Neither can we continue to take a silent stance on matters that compromise principles of moral integrity, lest we reap havoc on our very existence as a society and as a world.

The world's record of amoral conditions is conclusive in confirming that a decline in morality weakens societies. Unfortunately, this is our present course with matters of homosexuality. The part of our national focus that supports homosexuality as a viable lifestyle, for instance, is moving us to lower grounds of immorality. This ill-fated move has surfaced with assistance from elected officials who dare entertain homosexuality as a way of life to be decided by majority vote.

State or national enactment of such a plan compounds the matter of homosexuality with volumes of high risk potentials. The most immediate danger is disregard for the "Supreme Holder" of executive power who rules on all matters as the **Chief Executive** of majority and minority vote. His decision on the appropriateness of homosexuality was issued ages ago; "Thou shalt not lie with mankind, as womankind: it is abomination."[31] Therefore, by virtue of God's executive command, the effect of a popular or legislative vote that sanctions homosexuality as a rightful practice is a vote for sin. This makes the actual vote an act of indiscretion as well.

Public approval of homosexuality to the extent of legalizing same sex unions violates the sanctity of marriage between a man and woman. Moreover, it dishonors the natural institution of marriage and family. Popular support of homosexual practice also sends a dangerous message of encouragement to children. We run the risk of altering their purpose as the life line to future generations, thus diminishing our longevity as a society and as a world.

Beyond that impact, legalizing homosexuality as a rightful sex act is a public disservice, especially to members of the gay community. Not only is homosexuality sinful; two hundred years of concealment also makes it an abnormal act. Either way, the nature of men and women and the very purpose for which God created them are violated. Again, within the frame of our moral duty, there is a more appropriate need. Homosexuality is best classified as an illness that requires measures of behavioral modification, accordingly. This move would certainly be no more than our response to alcoholism and drug addiction, and it should be no less.

We have come a long way by God's grace and with a new attitude about life. In the more recent course of our journey, modern perceptions have changed our moral character in several respects. We have evolved to a time when man's word is seldom his bond. The golden rule is becoming a practice of doing unto others before they do unto us. Sometimes we forgive and sometimes we manage to forget, but many times our priority is to first get even.

In confusing matters of social inclusion and moral acceptance, we tend to angle our ears, eyes, hearts, and minds to tolerate almost every sin from A to Z. Common indiscretions that were formerly left in the proverbial closet of skeletons are now promoted on television and theater screens. Our modern liberated spirit permits players to move steadily beyond the point of sinning with shame to a time of being bold with sin. So far, we can estimate that our public support in response to homosexuality is one of the boldest moves that man has made against godliness.

These points are not stated with disregard for all of the good that we are and do as a society. They are reminders to reinforce the idea that our moral obligation requires us to recognize and respond to sin in any form of practice as sin. Therefore, we must be willing to retain ourselves as decisive and determined players in the task of upholding morals that are based on the laws of God. Otherwise, we run the risk of invoking the worst of God's wrath against us. The possible magnitude of that consequence is the greatest threat that we could ever experience in the game.

War jeopardizes our personal victory in the game of life. Nations have historically sought to protect their interests and prosperity. This task has evolved as a territorial matter of ownership and is pursued relentlessly by some nations as designated warfare. In the present decade, the United States has become the focus of international concern as a high risk target for military attack. Prevailing threats of this situation underline the second issue for this particular passage. The purpose is to review specific dynamics of war and peace in relationship to our moral character and purpose.

An overwhelming prophecy of war as recorded in the Players' Manual predicts a time when wars will cease.[32] Until that appointed time comes, war will continue as an inevitable deed of man's inhumanity that extracts the lowest form of barbarianism from civility. On an interpersonal level, it is easy to perceive war as an act of God, but regarding war in such a manner conflicts with God's nature of perfect peace. The fact that God is always in control of His creation and wills us peace provides an optional thought: war is a creation of man that God allows to happen.

Persistence in speculating reasons for God's decisions on this matter is inconsequential because the manual is precise in covering God's plan for war and peace. The Book of Ecclesiastes dictates a universal order and time for everything that happens under God's sun, thus affording a time for war and a time for peace.[33]

Since worldwide impacts of war are always relevant, players are in a position to make general assessments. From one perspective, for instance, our recent invasion of Iraq is perceived as an unwise and unsafe presidential call. Not only did the mission of finding weapons of mass destruction fail, the invasion has not proved successful as a means to world peace.

The mission of securing global peace ideally begins with two assertions. Players need to first realize that war begets war. The second point suggests that war is a misplay of perceptions. Both of these assertions take into consideration that war is triggered by different factors and occurs at every level of social existence in different ways. Not only are we at war with others, we are at war with ourselves as a nation and within ourselves as individuals.

Life is sometimes a grand mess because we are not in agreement on what God wants for and from all of His people. Worse than this situation, we are still at odds in our perceptions about the existence of God. This conflict heightens the risk of our individual and national existence because God is the permanent foundation of our moral system. Whenever we distance Him from any aspect of the human experience, our morals are bound to be slanted to our wants instead of His. These situations and others contribute to why our struggles toward world peace remain on he shallow end of success.

On the matter of war verses peace, the evidence of what God wants is clearly visible. His last public broadcast of a peace plan aired with the delivery of Jesus, the only universally proclaimed "Prince of Peace."[34] During His lifetime on earth, Jesus issued a verbal endorsement of God's peace plan, accordingly; "Blessed are the peacemakers: for they shall be called the children of God."[35] This endorsement naturally disqualifies warmongers from the same entitlement because their main strategy for peace is to huff and puff until they blow up the world.

Peace treaties, world alliances, and involvements of the United Nations are usually progressive steps toward world peace. In spite of these valued efforts, we will continue to fall short of our goal until nations rely on God as the ammunition and the bullet proof vest of life.

Meanwhile, there is yet another important reason that explains why the goal of world peace remains unaccomplished. From both an individual and national perspective, our instinctive concern in making concessions is that of self. The question is always the same: "What's in it for me?"

Whenever "self" is the main focus of pursuit, players tend to claim territorial rights without much thought about who holds the title of total ownership in the game. We claim ownership on all goods that we amass by any means until, for whatever reasons, they have no value or cease to exist. Usually, this normal perception of ownership is somehow re-directed when tragedy or death is the principal cause for our loss. We not only concede that God is the owner, we ascribe to "His will" being the reason for our loss.

During the fatal event of September 11th in 2001, the

world lost a big chunk of American cheese that totaled more than three thousand lives. Although the loss of that cheese created a major disruption in our lives, the more important point is that our ownership was and is always null and void. That particular cheese, as it is with all cheese, was owned by somebody else. Realization of the rightful owner became apparent in our immediate and swift U-turns to God for logic, solace, and the strength to endure.

September 11th, in effect, may have been a final wake-up call for us to make several moves from old habits. For all practical purposes, we need to move away from activating God as a temporary figurine of relief in times of personal, national, and worldwide crises. We must also make a move to upgrade our moral agenda to a level that facilitates our coexistence as one nation and one world under God.

Whether as a civilian or military force, we are first accountable to God. Therefore, our primary responsibility is to consult with Him before, during, and after we make our moves in life. Regardless of how significant or insignificant our actions may be, we must learn to manage life according to God's directives to us.

In contrast to the positive effects of obeying God, our tendency toward habitual disobedience is the most negative element of the human experience and the game. Since the time of Adam and Eve, our patterns of disobedience have not changed too much for the better. We constantly violate every rule in the manual. As we grow in stature, little fibs become perjury, spankings become death by lethal injection, and resentment becomes world wars.

The urgency for players to navigate life with God at the helm makes obedience to God a key factor in the quest for world peace. Though few in number, war-prone nations in the Middle East appear to be about as far from peaceful coexistence now as they probably were when beginning their conflicts. They have proven for centuries that war is what happens when leaders forget God. Securing peace may or may not have been among their initial motives for war, but the impact of war on peace is a vital consideration for the coexistence of all nations.

Prolonged episodes of warfare should confirm for lead players in the game that military combat is not a suitable means to peace. Yet, when the bait of military warfare was dangled before American eyes in 2001, the chief players made a move to find weapons of mass destruction. Until the present time, consequences of invading Iraq in 2002 have been costly in human lives, installments of various high-powered security systems, and continued warfare in a land freed from a brutal regime. There is also the undue burden of emotional and financial stress, the brunt of which is shouldered by America citizens. The most obvious point is that while a time for war and peace has been pronounced in the manual of life, the goal of pursuing peace does not present a time for war.

Whenever matters of war and peace are pursued without petitioning God for His countenance, players run the risk of living dangerously at the mercy of God. This situation parallels relationships among bosses and their employees and of married couples. In the case of children, living dangerously at the mercy of their parents is probably a way of life. Some teenagers run this risk when they miss their curfews without parental permission.

Failure to acknowledge God in all of our ways has great implications for world peace.[36] A significant risk is compromising the overall purpose of the game. God is not in the business of rewarding us for wars fought without His support. Therefore, for the sake of realizing world peace, we must first realize that peace is an outgrowth of brotherly love.

Inasmuch as Jesus taught that we should love our neighbors as ourselves, loving our fellowman is a moral obligation that is inherent to obeying God.[37] Peace, then, is a rationale for our obedience to God, the development of which begins at home.

An earnest intent on securing world peace should cause us to pray in the manner that Jesus prayed during the final hours of His purpose on earth, accordingly: not our will, but thine be done.[38] This intent also forces a need for us to give greater significance to human life as an extension of God. In missions of peace, we have neither the physical power to kill God nor His authority to kill mankind.

There is no doubt that players have a great number of conflicts to resolve in the interest of peace. Some are personal, social, and racial in origin. Some are related to family, job, and even church situations. Others have been contingent upon plans for securing world peace. All of these conflicts are common obstacles in the game, but some are more threatening than others.

The potential impact of recurring conflicts in pursuits for world peace is always a prevailing threat. Yet, the United States has enjoyed freedom from declared warfare on its soil since the Civil War ended in 1865. Our capable presence in achieving this luxury is hardly limited to human effort. The aftermath of September 11th is adequate proof that individual and national recovery is never successful by human effort alone.

Players rise above their pain and loss by God's will; and so it is with nations. We have managed possession of our war-free territory with the grace and aid of an "unchanging Hand" that should never be confused with the "good hands" commercialized by Allstate. The same relief is ever available for our peace missions. Our one option is to ask God for what we need, that being His directive. Whenever we ask with faith and obedience, we shall receive.[39]

The church is the permanent base of our moral values. All behaviors that we officially endorse or promote by tradition reflect various features of our character as a society. The moral aspect of our character develops from a combination of factors, beginning with home and school environments. Beyond these two centers of influence, the church has the broad responsibility of preserving our religious heritage by transmitting moral principles from one generation to the next.

More than any other social setting, the church is the primary learning center that is established specifically to equip us with the required capacity to win the game of life. However, as the world continues to evolve from the sanctity of principles and practices of the past, the move of the church from its primitive function is subject to debate. At the center of contention is the effectiveness of the church in meeting the moral needs of society as opposed to accommodating immoral trends. A review of this unsettling issue is the final presentation on moral foundations of the game.

Home team players have traditionally perceived and relied upon the church as the local establishment of religion that functions as a place where congregations grow in Christian morals. According to the experiences of a woman remembered from the neighborhood of my childhood, traditional and modern perceptions of the church may no longer be an ideal match.

71

My playmates and I were always amused whenever this woman raved about *almost* losing her religion. We were sympathetic and amused whenever we learned from her boastful reports that she had actually lost her religion. Eventually, instead of wishing for recovery of her lost religion, we concluded among ourselves that losing her religion was not too much of a big deal; seemingly, she always found her religion each time that it was lost. For a goodly while, we had no idea that she was losing her religion in the heat of anger. In fact, we had no earthly idea about how religion could be lost at all.

Several years after we became adults, an unthinkable situation happened. This same woman, by her account of events, finally lost all of her religion in church. She later changed her church membership and, after a brief time, stopped attending church altogether.

In retrospect, the case of anybody losing religion in church suggests three possibilities. Perhaps the church continues to be a local establishment of religion because it has become a place where religion is lost so often that it can be stacked in piles. If this is true, then it is possible that some religion has been lost in the church for reasons other than anger. Perhaps piles of lost religion are stored in churches because the spiritual climate is so filled with strife, corruption, confusion, and negative vibes, that the atmosphere is more typical of a war zone instead of a spiritual haven.

Given these possibilities, a reasonable concern is the extent to which the church is showing firmness or losing its footing as the seat from which moral ethics are cultivated. Any doubt about this specific mission further implicates social change as a tremendous weight in the game of life.

When Jesus Christ was commissioned to establish

the church, God had already designed its purpose to with-stand even the gates of hell; and so it will.[40] However, in that purpose, the natural course of change was not to be altered; the most obvious reason being that change is God's course of time and His choice of plan. Thus, the history of organized religion reveals that the church is certainly no exception as a target of social change.

Change in the Christian Church has been prominent since the Great Schism in 1054 that divided the Christian world into the Roman Catholic and Greek Orthodox Churches. Later, in the early years of the sixteenth century, Martin Luther and John Calvin were the two principal players in the game whose influence led to the Protestant Reformation. Much of this movement was based on religious doctrine in conjunction with political authority, but moral issues also dominated. One of the most notorious events of the Reformation era was England's break with the Roman Catholic Church under the rule of King Henry VIII (ca 1520). Thereafter, the Anglican Church emerged in part to accommodate marriage among clergy, divorce, and to improve acceptance of royal heirs born outside of the Roman Catholic Church.[41]

Morality is not a competition. In 1563, the Church of England began official Protestant operations as the Anglican Church.[42] Since that time, organized religion expanded throughout the world with a great number of Protestant denominations. Though each is based on selective principles and practices of Christian doctrine, some are now struggling to maintain a sense of Christian purpose. A part of this struggle is the apparent need to function effectively amidst changes in a modern world.

The rapid pace of social change in more recent times is almost forcing the church to be much more immediate in fulfilling its purpose. While responding to this urgency, some church congregations are more focused on competing against each other. This unassigned agenda of the church may have a bit of merit, be it ever so temporary. Nevertheless, in the balance of common purpose, the internal character of many local churches is still overweight in some instances and underweight in others.

Overweight characters tend to be overwhelming in their ministries. So much is going on within the same time frame that little is being accomplished by way of spiritual or moral enhancement. The church mission and related programs are overshadowed by attempts to adopt as much as possible from worship services and additional program features of other churches. As a result, the character of these competitive churches lingers in a state of confused identity. The church itself loses all sense of its traditional perspective.

Churches with an underweight character are so cold in nature that their best appeal to the public is anemic in passion, commitment, service, and leadership. Most members do not know each other and the minister hardly knows the members. These are the basic one-day-a-week Sunday churches.

Regardless of the character generated by church memberships, churches are the moral headquarters of the world. Without changing Christian doctrine, the church ministry is always expected to reflect an inner and outer image of Christian discipline. Inasmuch as Christian culture changes, as does the world, church ministries need to be modified only to expand the pursuit of Christian purposes while preserving Christian principles.

Unfortunately, some individual church programs are so far off course in their missions that congregations often fail or miss opportunities to be productive in society as well as in local communities. Instead of these organized systems of Christianity transforming the world, they risk being transformed by the world. The greatest weakness is a lack of moral decorum.

Whether or not members are engaged in worship, business sessions, or related activities, all kinds of behavior are not suitable for sustaining hallowed grounds. The point is not to suggest excluding members and visitors from church attendance on the basis of their behavior; quite the contrary. If a common nature of man is to behave according to where he is at a given time, then home team players must assure that the church can, indeed, be recognized as a church by its sacred atmosphere and Christian outreach. This action is inherent to expanding the kingdom of God on earth.

Ultimately, the character of a church is the strength and weakness of leadership and membership. As such, the task of being relevant and effective in a changing world requires interpersonal relationships between and among clergy and laity to be morally sound in principle and practice.

In the same respect, if congregations are to gain future longevity as a positive influence in society, the church mission must be pursued with moral sensibility. Prior to "dressing up" the internal character for public appeal, a mere desire or perceived need for change is not sufficient for effective and meaningful change. There must be moral maturity to ensure that change is implemented without tarnishing Christian ideals.

Occasionally, regardless of how urgent a need for change may be, the task of gaining support is not always easily managed. The mere forethought of change can be risky business, especially with the involvement of old established congregations.

Church members are known for sticking to the idea,

"If it ain't broke, don't fix it," when it would be more beneficial to realize that if it [the church] ain't growing, it's broke! Sometimes, the need to upgrade outreach ministries and other church operations are delayed so long that change is either forced, too late, or not feasible at all. Least of all should congregations oppose program enhancement just because "it has been that way for fifty years."

Obviously, fifty years is a reputable age in the life of a church, but only if it has been productive over fifty years. Modern times make it easier for older congregations to become boring and stagnated to the point of losing their appeal. In turn, there may be far more decline than growth in the number of their members.

In the context of "aging gracefully," institutional maturity among congregations and denominations enables tolerance of opposing views without consequences of any minister or church member being threatened, penalized, or isolated. Clergy and lay are better able to face challenging truths and problems and, together, purge the system with change in harmonious spirit. Moral maturity is satisfying Christian responsibility by processing the standard mission of the church in a changing society for the purpose of Christian unity.

God does not authorize players to change the mission of the church. Popularity of mega-churches in the American experience has slightly influenced a migratory move from denominational worship to interfaith worship. As younger generation players find their niche in a new wave of passionate worship, traditional congregations are left with the task of refining their church programs. Some may need to reform their internal character in a way that does not cause members to lose their religion or compel them to change or terminate their membership. Maybe old feuds among members or between them and the minister(s) need to be settled once and for all. Perhaps there are matters of internal corruption that need to be resolved once and for all. Failure to do so can only result in established players submitting to a newness in the tradition of church life that may or may not be effective.

Reality of that thought returns us to the same song, third verse: if the character of a church ain't effective, then it's broke!

The overriding potential of modernizing tradition may prove risky in the long haul of the church mission. Specifically stated, shouting hosannas in a mammoth "high praise" worship service may have a value of worship, but not necessarily a value of committed faith. If this potential proves to be real, then the goal of moral enhancement will be even more difficult to accomplish.

Regardless of what the church setting eventually becomes, it will never escape being a target of change. Neither will the church ever be destroyed by the impact of a changing world. But the fact that social change is inevitable makes transition a key element in finalizing adjustments.

Smooth transition between the old and new depends on a number of individual and group factors that include attitudes, commitment to change, and diplomacy. Whenever change involves a broad field of options, ideas must be appealing before they are accepted. In a scheme of forcing ideas, players do not take too kindly to being coerced or railroaded into propositions or final decisions.

Silent resistance is known to be a powerful prelude to public revolt. For this reason, in continued efforts of reforming the world from a Christian perspective, the home team cannot afford to impose Christian doctrine or values.

The consequences of forced decisions also tend to weaken and often destroy enthusiasm and support. In such a case, our moral purpose in the game, though never itself perfected, stands a chance of becoming further fragmented by the opposition.

There is no evidence of Jesus influencing change in ways other than by peaceful means. Even with His final breath while nailed to a cross, Jesus influenced change by the example of His life. He remains the ageless model of moral reform. Therefore, for the church at large to continue transforming the world from moral irresponsibility, this task is better pursued with our lives on the line as examples of Christian principles.

Of all the moves made by the home team in pursuing the Christian mission of the church, the internal character, climate, and program are the full extent of what can be changed in the process. We must understand clearly that the church was established to represent the life and ministry of Jesus Christ.[43] The ordained emphasis assigned as the mission of the church, therefore, is never to be altered because Jesus Himself is the very foundation of the church. The choice of changing this predestined plan is not of human will, purpose, or pursuit.

Aside, from God's grace, our primary means to longevity as a Christian society resides in the youth of our churches. As we strategize to meet the challenges of a changing world, let us not move too far from "ATOZEE." Beyond this need of caution, let us not move too far from God and our moral responsibility to obey His laws.

In our performance as a church, while we persist in duplicating tutorial functions of formal education systems, let us focus more on teaching our youth the way of

Christianity. While we attempt to accommodate their diversified interests, let us attract them to the way of Christianity. While we allow them flexibility in their religious views, let us show them the way of Christianity. Above all else, let us constantly tell and remind them of the "ageless story" about an "ageless Man" with an "ageless name," from His manger to an "ageless rugged cross," and from His Ascension to heaven to His spiritual abode in human hearts.

On Your Mark, Get Set, . . . Not Yet! (Personal Foundations of the Game)

Five of every ten married players are probably guilty of one specific mental crime: they forget special days such as Valentine's Day or their wedding anniversary. Other players probably recall times when they remembered these special occasions with barely enough time to save face. Even if the second situation is a onetime incident, it is one of many that causes us to experience a mental shock of "last-minute unreadiness."

Episodes of last-minute unreadiness are frequent enough to be a standard way of life in the human experience. These are extremely brief and isolated periods of time when, during any quarter of the game, players suddenly remember to do or say something before it's too late.

Last-minute memory tasks are just as common among children as they are among adults. Children who misjudge the whereabouts of their parents make quick attempts to cover up their involvement in some "prohibited" activity. In their haste, they usually fail to remove all leading evidence from view. Invariably, upon hearing their parents getting closer to the scene, they make a last-minute dash to remove any remaining piece of evidence to escape punishment.

Many of us as grocery shoppers can identify with being in the check-out line before remembering a particular item that we also intended to purchase. There is also the episode of remembering to turn off the lights or stove within one step of leaving home. A classic seasonal episode is remembering at the last minute to hide a special Christmas gift that we intend to present as a great surprise.

Regardless of how late we may remember to do a "must do" task or how long we are delayed by taking care of last-minute urgencies, seldom do these episodes interfere with our plans or schedules. Somehow, we usually manage to buy a gift at the last minute and still arrive at the airport in time to make a scheduled flight. Getting to work on time under the same pressure is probably another story. Clearly indicated, situations vary in circumstances.

Occasionally, there are occurrences of last-minute episodes when the matter at hand does not require immediate action. These cases allow us the choice of responding later or not at all. However, when we rely on situations to resolve themselves, we set ourselves up for regrets and guilt trips.

Unforeseen circumstances have a way of making first and second chances impossible. Often are the times when some of us wish that we had acted on our last-minute impulses. Such a case is common among family members who, because of pure stubbornness, refuse to apologize for mistreating each other.

Procrastination and shifting of priorities are also factors that have a lot to do with us being too late in life. Students who forego a last-minute need to study for an exam usually suffer the consequences of being too late. They put themselves in a position to fail. More often than we want, failure is sometimes final.

Of all the situations that players experience in life, one in particular does not allow even half a moment for us to have an episode of last-minute unreadiness. Least of all is there time to take care of some forgotten detail at the last minute, regardless of how urgent the matter may be. As little as we may care to think about it, that situation would be our departure from the game.

At the exact time of a player's scheduled exit from the game of life, there is no opportunity to create an alibi, beg, stall, or negotiate for more time. Hence, a chance to make last-minute amends or to make up time wasted is totally non-existent. Whenever our personal game is over, it's over!

Nothing is incidental about God and human life. Every occurrence in the human experience happens with God's knowledge and by His power. Just as we never knew when we would be born, we know neither the day nor hour of our scheduled departure from the game; only God knows.[44] Our primary advantage is having the choice to live each day in final preparation for the eternal journey that, indeed, we will take one day. Inasmuch as the destination of that journey is always determined by God, our earthly existence is no more than a big class in life that we take. We must pass the class in order to win the game of life.

Every course that students take between elementary school and college has pre-established goals that students are expected to meet. In satisfying these goals, students are required to perform certain tasks with proficiency. The quality of their overall performance, however, is the main criterion that determines whether they pass or fail the course. Our existence between birth and death in the class of life follows that same pattern. Since we are not even close to being perfect, many a player probably gets into heaven with a "D" average. The goal is not to have an "F" average in the final minute.

The goal that all players are expected to accomplish is predetermined by God; that being the promotion of our souls from earth to heaven. Any chance that we may have of spending eternity with Him depends on how well we perform the primary task of loving Him with faith and obedience. Thus, our overall performance is one that requires and improves with spiritual growth.

Players have only the first quarter to grow into physical adulthood, and all of their physical adulthood to reach spiritual adulthood. Since the second quarter marks the beginning of our physical adulthood, it is also the designated time for players to decide the manner in which they will play the game and to assume full responsibility for their performance.

Players who are genuinely interested in winning the game must be willing to accept the identity of being a "peculiar" people.[45] This primary step requires commitment to God through faith in Jesus Christ and earnest attempts to comply with the ideals of Christian living on a daily basis.

Whether or not we are concerned about our post-game fate at all, the game of life is a natural challenge that can be extremely difficult if players are not properly anchored in Jesus. This likelihood draws attention to the fact that the game is an intense competition between God and Satan's teams, and has been so since the creation of mankind. The more that some players commit themselves to do God's will, the more they may find themselves tempted to do otherwise. This situation is common in the game because Satan works through all players to plot against God and His purpose. Satan's persistence and deceptive influence in the game are two main factors that make it important for home team players to choose their deeds, paths, and friends wisely.

In spite of our health and wealth or the kind of player that we choose to be, the game of life is not the easiest contact sport to play. All players receive bruises of some kind before leaving the game. Yet, whatever our experiences may be, we can always find inner peace and strength in the reality of knowing God through faith. He avails Himself to us and makes it possible for us to reach Him in a variety of ways, including through music, psychiatrists, and television.

With this diverse accessibility to Him, we should readily understand that God is far from being an isolated concept of spirituality. His presence is always directly behind and in front of us, and to the right and left side of us. There is no way that we can miss Him. However, achieving a meaningful relationship with Him is a matter of how personal we allow Him to be in our lives, individually and collectively.

Of our many assets in life, the omnipotence of God's presence is one of the greatest assets that we have in the game. As we grow closer to God in faith, His love for us becomes more obvious. We find ourselves relying more often on the power of His love because He is always whatever and wherever we need Him to be on the good side of life. As our "spiritual Parent," God is the only one who patiently tolerates all of our sins while making provisions for our basic needs. Never does He wait until the last minute to send sunshine or rain; neither does He ever respond to any of our needs by incident.

Players habitually overlook the fact that God takes care of the entire world. Out of the pureness of His love and power, He is on call to many billions of people twenty-four hours every day. This service is in addition to all of the other great things that He does to accommodate our personal and worldly comfort. He omits nothing in the process. Yet His unblemished record of response to us is never enough. We constantly gripe about something, especially the weather; it's either too cold or too hot.

Perhaps, the greatest flaw that we find in God is His slowness. He never fails to address our needs, but His responses are not always as quick as we expect or desire them to be. After all, we have evolved as a world of players who rely on instant gratification.

In proper context, any time that God appears to be slow or late, we have only ourselves to blame. Once we contact God for His help, some of us await His delivery with great anxiety. Many other players, because they misinterpret God's love, tend to clock Him with desperate measures and impatient pleas; "God, drop whatever you're doing and come see about me NOW!" They seek His relief fairly much in the same way of requesting services from any repairman. But these players aren't totally alone in their moments of desperation. Others of us, in our wayward human logic, also expect problems that are three years in the making to be solved within a few hours, if not seconds.

Only among the "peculiar" breed of players is there understanding of what it means to "Rest in the Lord, and wait patiently for Him."[46] This level of understanding underlines the meaning of what spiritual growth is all about; it maximizes our ability to attain inner peace and strength from the veil of God's grace.

Essentially, we grow to the point of realizing and accepting the fact that God is always in control of His purpose and ours. Then, at some higher level of faith, we learn that God's control is never incidentally programmed. Because He reigns forever, there will always be a season for everything and an exact time for His divine purpose to be fulfilled.

According to a specific hymn of faith, God's overall response of love to us validates His presence in the game as "our Maker, Defender, Redeemer, and Friend." With that kind of relationship going on, what more could any player ever need in the game of life? One thing for sure, there is no greater love than the love of God!

God rules the good, bad, ugly, and whatever else we choose to become during the game. Along with our special effects and defects, all players are born with potential to reach a certain point in life. Some of us become mothers and fathers, but not necessarily parents because we lack the potential. Players who actually become parents may be among the most charitable people in existence; many are not even biological bearers of children.

Parents maintain a spiritual endowment of invisible eyes and ears, strategically positioned to inform them of most things that their children do and say. Parents are also the mothers and fathers who love, nourish, and protect their young until releasing them onto the stage of adulthood. At this point of release, while many of these parents hang up their rights and privileges as disciplinarians, they continue their presence of love and support.

This particular release in the life of earth-parents is not featured in the parental reign of God. His rights and privileges as our Father are supreme and, by His choice and power, they are also permanent. As His children, the conditions of our purpose prohibit our ability to terminate His parental control over us. Yet, much to His displeasure, we choose to ignore His governance as children so often choose to ignore the authority of their earth-parents. We do sin, don't we?

86

Consequential to our choice in this respect is one prevailing thought. God is skilled in making His parental presence known to players who reject His supremacy as well as He does to those who accept His authority. The tragedy of September 11th is a memory that proves this point. That same event is one of an endless number that reflects His parental sacrifice. God reveals Himself in rescue missions as much as He does in other wonders of the game.

When God sees fit, He can force our obedience and love, but He usually accommodates our mix of choices with a great deal of patience. His preference is for us to accept, love, and obey Him on our own because that is our purpose in relationship to His overall existence. Beyond this thought are three other realities to be considered in conjunction with our purpose in the game, beginning with the creation of mankind.

God's initial design of human purpose was for man to "be fruitful, and multiply, and replenish the earth. . . ."[47] This was His first commandment of social order. Given the most recent census bureau count, the order to "multiply" may be the least difficult for players to obey.

Regardless of reasons involved, the failure of players to have children is never in conflict with God's purpose; neither are the brutal circumstances under which many babies are born and, sometimes, die. As unfortunate as these situations are, they are also designed to serve God's purpose in the human experience.

Secondly, there is but one living God, and we will never become Him or be as powerful as He is. Satan has tried since his appearance on earth and fails in that mission every day. His moves to undermine the existence, supreme nature, and purpose of God are as active now as when he enticed Eve to eat fruit from the "tree of knowledge" against God's will.[48] Other biblical reports of Satan's notorious determination include the case of Job's trials and tribulations. In that situation, Satan's influence rubbed off on Job's nagging wife, who also persisted unsuccessfully for Job to curse God.[49]

The fact that God created us in His image removes nothing from the reality that man will never have the capacity of God.[50] Even the fact that God ranks us just "a little lower than the angels" of heaven does not suggest that possibility; naturally, it wouldn't. The superiority of God's thoughts and ways is nowhere near being the same as ours.[51] These and all other differences between God and man clearly translate into the dominance of His perfection over our imperfection.

When God assigned players the privileges of serving as stewards of His property, we became the "intelligencia" of His earthly kingdom. He gave us "dominion over the fish of the sea, and over the fowl of the air, and over every living thing that moveth upon the earth. . . ."[52] This assignment sealed the highest position that we are to ever have on God's behalf during the game.

Our stewardship has little to do with living an affluent life. This has been the case ever since Adam and Eve were evicted from the Garden of Eden. Their sins could also be the reason why so many of us will never sail the high seas on a yacht catered with champagne. Interestingly enough, blaming Adam and Eve's disobedience for our lack of wealth and luxurious comfort is not altogether ridiculous.

Players who tend to fault others for their limitations and misfortunes in the game would have no problem holding the first man and lady of Eden responsible. They would probably suggest that if Adam and Eve had just left "the tree" alone, maybe our journey in life would be much less complicated. The truth of this matter is we have not seen the half of what could be worse. Nevertheless, in all of the many centuries gone by, players have been no less disobedient.

The history of our sinfulness can surely be traced to the time of Adam and Eve, but not restricted to their downfall in life. We can only hold ourselves responsible for our sinful behavior in the game. The reality of each player not owning a yacht or being in a position to enjoy the finest luxuries of life is simple to understand. God's design of human purpose is not intended for our circumstances and experiences to be the same. By His choice, each of us is a different individual whose individual path in life has been chartered according to our differences. Thus, the design of our character weighs heavily on our performance in the game.

In our evolution from households to nations, various patterns of our coexistence eventually dictated a need for organized leadership. As a result, we have heads of states and designated "heads of households" for income tax purposes. God's ability to foresee the social spread of human conduct reasonably accounts for why He has never deputized man to perform on His behalf as a sovereign being. Had this delegation of authority taken place, heaven would surely be a place scarce in number. The fact that we do not have God's capacity makes His complete design and assessment of human purpose another asset in the game.

The matter of who has and who owns sovereignty in the game is indisputable. Whereas we have been entrusted with the responsibility of God's landed estate, there is nothing absolute or permanent about man's authority in the world. God empowered us as His stewards of earth, and He can strip us of that power at will and at any time.

God, and only God, rules the world and mankind. If truth be admitted, we do not really want to know or even imagine what His world would be otherwise. Since our hearts, minds, and tongues get us into trouble so much, the idea of man's absolute rule is extremely frightening. Barbaric leadership styles practiced by Saddam Hussein and others of uncivilized character are even more frightening. Then, too, there is the matter of chaos and corruption stemming from the management of our homes, schools, and churches.

Amidst our on-going trends of civil and criminal disorder, the same consolation prevails. In none of our social domains does any man have absolute governance. Furthermore, God always keeps everything in divine order. Therefore, "let us not be weary in well-doing: for in due season we shall reap, if we faint not."[53]

All things considered, our authoritative entitlement has led us to do good things and things that are not so good. In our personal strides, we have made phenomenal discoveries and progress in all walks of life. We have also made some heavy-duty mistakes. Perhaps the most critical evidence of our earthly stewardship suggests that while we please God in so many different ways, we also continue to irritate and disappoint Him in just as many different ways.

The fact that God created the world and everything therein reinforces the reality of why He holds the ultimate plan for and of man's purpose. He also has innate power of attorney over all mankind and anything that we so daringly believe is formed by our ingenuity. Keeping this thought in mind, we should be content to awaken each new day with the knowledge that our lives are contained in God's purpose.

Whether or not God created mankind because of loneliness does more than rekindle the matter of "what was God thinking?" The proof that He created us, already knowing our shortcomings, just reinforces the reality that God can handle everything that He creates. Confirmations of His energy are infinite in number.

We must remember that the two most important and dramatic events in the history of man's existence were not caused by man. Jesus was born and crucified amidst hate, fear, and other insecurities; but each event happened by God's choice of purpose for mankind.

Beliefs that deny the existence of God and His supremacy as creator and ruler of all things are pathetically weak, but potent enough to contaminate our performance in the game. As a consequence, some players fall by the wayside and choose to stay down because they live without purpose. Specifically, they ignore God. The third reality of our purpose, therefore, justifies the need for us to "fix" our eyes upon Jesus; God placed Him as the centerpiece of human life. Without this focus, players can never experience the value of having a meaningful relationship with God.

Regardless of our final destination, the first step of our journey into eternity begins with the race of life that we run on earth. Our focus on God, or the lack thereof, establishes our "mark" for the race. Upon entering the second quarter, if not earlier, our choice is to run the race with or without Jesus in our lives. 'Tis a far better race to run with Jesus, side by side.

By God's calendar of human life, the playing time of man on earth is extremely brief, but always sufficient for accomplishing God's purpose. In the brief time that we have, running backward and forward in the game sets us up for severe consequences. If we fear going to hell at all, then we really cannot afford to do a lot of straddling while engaging in a relationship with God.

It is not uncommon, however, for players to make a sincere commitment to God late in the game; and that's a good move. Going to heaven is probably a miracle for most players. So the worst that we could ever do in the game is to never run the race with faith.

Every player has an ark to build. The race that we run in the game of life is as exciting or as dull as the moves we make. The benefits that we receive depend on how secure we are in the godly purpose of life. In symbolic terms, the success that we manage to experience depends on how well we choose to build our personal arks.

When God commanded Noah to build an ark in preparation for the Flood, the dimensions of the ark were extremely significant. They were ordered to accommodate a specific number of all living things for forty days and forty nights.[54]

Arks made by players for the game are of a much different order. Fashioned by the core of each player's heart and mind, the arks that we build represent our total presence in the game. They are repositories of everything that God decides and allows us to do or say throughout the game. Ideally, any design that we choose should direct, moralize, and energize our character and efforts as we seek to do the will of God. It should also be able to secure us on the stormy seas and just as much when we are safely housed on the calm shores of life.

The quality of these accommodations in our lives varies according to our choice of tools and materials. In the world of construction, we would not expect an urban dwelling to be built of straw or another to be erected with

92

mud piles and scotch tape. Likewise, we cannot build a life of love with hate, or one of respect with disrespect, or another of good with evil. These limitations in crafting our personal lives must be carefully considered as we "get set" on the mark from which we choose to play the game.

Among other preliminaries in declaring our design is the need to distinguish between our overall purpose and mission(s) in the game. God establishes our purpose and defines it by His laws. As a part of that process, our missions are whatever we choose to pursue under God's control. For instance, in cases of resolving social conflict, peace should always be our godly pursuit. However, and for whatever reasons, if we must choose war, then God allows us to fight until He gets tired and says, "Stop!"

Since God allows our missions to be based more on our personal preferences, they either help or hinder us in playing the game. The world is full of traps. So we need to be careful to not underestimate the consequences of life when the nature of our missions is deliberately and far removed from God's purpose for us. The selection of such missions is the same as demanding God to have mercy on us, rather than living in His grace. The same demand is in effect whenever we direct our deeds with evil intentions instead of with intentions of good will. In any event, God uses all of our choices, be they right, wrong, or different.

Short of possibly causing us to spend eternity in hell, our persistence in wrongdoing is bound to provoke the worst of God's wrath and indignation against us on earth. While this matter is worth additional consideration, the greater benefit is for us to focus on the *promised* consequences of our pursuits when they involve missions that are pleasing to God. To manage this task effectively requires clarity in how we perceive and accept the reality of God's intervention during the course of our missions.

All players have routine and specific jobs to do for God. In making His special assignments, God sometimes designates many players for the same particular job, but plans a different way for each player to get the job done. For this reason, He develops us with different potentials and a capacity that either allows or rejects flexibility in our attitudes, habits, talents, and other distinguishing features.

Every player has a different story to tell and, of all the many blind players in the world, each has a unique way of seeing the same world.

More than the design of our arks, the building process reflects the quality of our daily performance throughout the game. The type of tools and materials that we develop or choose in life for this ongoing effort varies according to our commitment or lack of commitment to God.

With the beginning of each generation or class in life, the world is potentially populated with do-gooders and evildoers, the rich and poor, and the healthy and unhealthy. As we progress in the human experience, the reality of what we become proves that new players are not necessarily confined to the background of their birth or native character. We often notice, for instance, that all big babies do not become big adults in size, nor do all strong players remain strong.

In the same frame of thought, there are times when we limit our progress by our tendency to speculate the future of human possibilities on averages derived from statistical probabilities instead of God's all-time abilities. One basic difference between God and man is the fact that God manages all aspects of human activity with absolute precision. He also controls all probabilities. Therefore, our lifestyles, missions, and all else connected to human existence can be altered if God so chooses. His range of choice and change in our lives even includes the purpose that He has already established for us by His laws.

Another relevant point is our individual missions are not totally defined within the range of our circumstances or by the level of persistence with which we pursue our choices. Our lives and our missions are always under the control of God. Therefore, He is at liberty to work His purpose through our missions as He sees fit, anywhere and at any time.

This perspective clarifies the position that nothing was incidental about the Flood or about Noah building an ark. Neither was anything incidental about Moses freeing a captive people from Pharaoh's army. God had a purpose that He directed in each of these instances. Furthermore, the verbal presence of God should be sufficient in dismissing any notion of incidental occurrence.

According to many individual missions documented in the manual, direct communication between God and man was once commonplace, but modified with the crucifixion of Jesus. Since the time of that event, our spiritual sense has been the vehicle through which God chooses to express His presence, though He continues to contact us through our ears, eyes, hearts, and minds. On any given day, we can detect His presence in wind-blown trees or just as much when we kneel in prayer.

The fact stands that we may or may never know God's designs on missions that we choose to pursue in life. Conversations during the last supper of Christ with His disciples add validity to this connection between God and human purpose.

Upon announcing that He would be betrayed by one of them, Jesus caused a major stir of curiosity among the disciples. Each of them wondered to the extent of asking,

"Lord, is it I?"[55] Judas, pretending to be naturally surprised, was probably tense with guilt; and well he should have been. There was no need for his astonishment. Because of financial greed, he was already involved in a plot against Jesus that aided the crucifixion of Jesus.

Peter's case varied a bit. He was known to be firm in boasting his love for Jesus and loyalty to Him. Totally unaware of his personal weakness, Peter seriously protested the prophetic claim that he would deny Jesus. Yet, at the most crucial time appointed by God, His purpose for Peter was fulfilled; Peter denied Jesus in the exact number of times that Jesus had cited.[56]

In the few days that followed, Thomas, another disciple, presented another kind of situation. While encountering Jesus face to face after Jesus arose from the grave, Thomas needed absolute proof that Jesus had, indeed, risen and was alive. Thomas was eventually free of his doubt, but only after being allowed to touch the wounded side of Jesus.[57]

From the Garden of Eden, through the earth-time of Jesus, to the present day, we can determine that the basic nature of man has not changed. Judases still live everywhere on the planet Earth, but so does God. His divine nature remains unchanged. Yet, some of us are no better than Thomas in our faith; nor are we any better than Peter and Judas in our love. We, too, fold under pressure. We also need absolute proof to convince us that there is a God who rules the universe and who knows our strengths as well as our weaknesses. The sun that shines upon us or the air that we breathe is never sufficient.

Whatever beliefs, disbeliefs, or doubts that we may or may not have about the existence of God and His almighty power are not incidental to God. They revert to His plan of purpose for each of us. Whenever we are moved to demand or debate evidence of God in any respect of His true nature, the situation itself is a test of our faith. Furthermore, it reflects the overall quality of our arks.

If winning the game is to be our top priority, then we must concede that faith is the only factor in our human experience that makes the benefits of God's promises possible:[58]

The poor in spirit shall gain access to heaven.

The mourners shall be comforted.

The meek shall inherit the earth.

The hungry and thirsty shall be filled.

The merciful shall obtain mercy.

The pure in heart shall see God.

The peacemakers shall be called children of God.

The persecuted shall be entitled to heaven.

Beyond these provisions, if we are consistently responsible to God, we have His promise of eternal life.[59]

Given these and many other guarantees in the game, our urgency should be removing ourselves from doubt and disbelief to a stable level of faith in God and His purpose. Whether or not we make this move our choice, we can be assured that nothing will ever be incidental about the manner in which we must live or choose to live.

Regardless of the manner that God allows us to live, He can enable or disable our missions. As He works His purpose through us, every player becomes a relevant example of something in the human experience. Be that example good or evil, the final result of our performance in the game depends on the strength of our faith in God through Jesus Christ. The dying thief who hung on a cross next to Jesus confirms this point; he went to heaven.[60]

Faith is our highest option in the game. In the world of tennis, failure to use specific equipment can result in players losing the game, set, and match. Such a loss parallels the game of life. Of all the tools and materials available for playing the game of life, some are more crucial than others. Without proof of having ever used three tools in particular, we automatically lose everything: the mark, game, and crown of eternal life.

Players who are extremely rigid in their assessment of God's requirements may be quick to identify faith as the only key to heaven. On the surface, this debatable position omits the interactions or chain effects of faith, hope, and love. In detailing this triage, we recall that Apostle Paul was emphatic in declaring love as the greatest feature of human character. This powerful declaration presents several noteworthy implications regarding our purpose in the game.

Regardless of team preference, all players need to know that God is a jealous God.[61] As a means of attracting our attention, it is His nature to challenge our love on the basis of our faith. He also challenges our faith on the basis of our love. In this respect, faith and love are inseparable; yet faith denotes the manner in which we perceive God, and our love denotes the range of our willingness to act for Him or on His behalf.

The story of Job captures this distinction and, at the same time, reveals the demanding nature of God. It further shows how strong we need to be in our commitment to Him. Through all the emotional trauma and physical pain that God allowed Job to suffer, Job remained quite clear and determined in the mission of fulfilling his purpose to God. In addition to Job's life being a testament of faith and love, it was a specific test of personal endurance to prove the power of faith. In the context of spiritual strength and momentum, God's purpose was to use Job's life as an example of enduring faith, hope, and love for our benefit.

When compared to faith and hope, love sustains our faith and provides us a firm base of hope. This is the kind of love that God expects from us. Consequently, we can definitely conceive love as being in the crop of tools that moves us in the direction of heaven's gates. Yet, if God is to be the central focus in our lives, we must first believe or have faith in Him as evidence of our love for Him. Otherwise, the hope of heaven becoming our eternal home has no sense of value.

At this point, we can reasonably speculate that hope builds and reinforces the spiritual momentum and strength of our faith. Therefore, in the absence of hope, any intention that players have about winning the game would be based on a false sense or spirit of faith, if not undiluted vanity. Some players are now bold enough that they would actually dare God to send them to hell.

The composite effect of faith, hope, and love enhances our performance from one quarter through the next. A rank order of significance in the value of these properties is a difficult assignment. Each of the three is indispensable when it comes to our purpose in life. However, with the least of assessments, faith is a must-have tool for playing the game because it sets us on the "mark to God." Hope and love are supportive tools that create and retain a balance of our faith and deeds once we get set for the race of life. They minimize the devil's interference in God's business.

On this basis, faith is a function of our love and hope that regulates our personal relationship with God. We can best capitalize on this emphasis by playing the game according to the following principles:

If we believe in God, then we should have faith in His presence.

If we believe that God has all power in His hands, then we should have faith in His sovereignty.

If we believe that God is the giver of all good and perfect gifts, then we should have faith in Jesus as our Lord and Savior.

If we believe in the Word of God, then we should have faith in His promise of eternal life.

If we believe that Jesus lives, then we should have faith in the power of His blood to make us whole.

The value of faith in the game has never been fully reconciled among players because of misconceived notions and problems in sifting rational thought from symbolic concepts. Despite provisions of biblical truths, some old issues just never die. Still unsettled in the mix of confusion is the "born again" concept, a familiar topic often associated with Nicodemus. In response to this matter, Jesus stated, "Except a man be born of water and of the spirit, he cannot enter into the kingdom of heaven."[62]

The modern focus of that same issue is no longer just the process; the amount of water is also a controversial matter. In the hope of unraveling mistaken notions, three points come to mind. First, baptism is a ritual that symbolizes a beginning or renewal of personal commitment to God and Christian doctrine. Secondly, faith is the reality of our beliefs and actions while engaged in that commitment. Thirdly, the belief that diving head-on into a pool of water or being sprinkled with drops of water from the river of Jordan is a free pass to heaven approaches spiritual insanity.

Nicodemus appears to have been sincere in his quest for understanding, but questioning biblical matters with sincerity is not always the case among players. Some of us debate the Bible for an unattached pleasure of social amusement, pleased with self-made and ungodly analyses of certain contents. Efforts of this kind should not be a routine of personal faith. Nevertheless, players of faith who engage in such spiritual trivia usually defend their beliefs with a margin of sensibility.

Players should strive to be "conceptually correct" with clarity when interpreting matters of Christian thought. As an example of applying symbolic logic to biblical concepts, being born again can be equated to going from rags to riches. Each concept shares the same implication of going from one state of life to a better or higher quality of life. However, without any degree of interpretation, the bare expression of either concept omits the much needed spiritual perspective of being born again.

Jesus, the Master Teacher of life, always taught from a spiritual perspective. Therefore, the task of grasping and accepting spiritual concepts requires us to expand our spiritual horizon with God through His Word and our faith. Until players grow in this direction, spiritual trivia will never cease.

Doubts and misconceptions that rouse biblical issues are also difficult to remove or correct because, quite often, we base biblical concepts on physical perspectives that have no possibility for physical reality. For example, reproducing man from a scoop of dust is humanly impossible, but if God ever chooses, He could easily reproduce man from a box of instant cake mix. He demonstrated this extent of His power through Jesus, who fed more than five thousand with two fishes and five loaves of bread.[63]

Players who lack unconditional faith in God cannot handle biblical truths. They will never accept the fact that the birth of Jesus was neither accidental nor incidental. The fact that He was conceived by a virgin is even more far-fetched. For these players, God's choice for Jesus to be born of a virgin and the reality of His birth being accomplished by God's power are biblical mysteries in need of scientific proof. Whenever scientific reason is impossible or inadequate, any mysterious move of God is labeled as an untruth; "it never happened. . . ." This was Pharaoh's mind-set until his army drowned in the Red Sea.

Pharaoh's downfall left a compelling message for all future generations of players. God did not create us to make His power official or worthy of belief. Our purpose, in this respect, is to acknowledge and rely on His power through faith without a need for justification. Furthermore, we must believe that God's power is the dominating force of all events and of all human existence. Thus, He intervenes in our lives and our purposes at will. These beliefs are basic to being born again.

In the game of life, the concept of being born again denotes a spiritual birth by which we seal our earthly union with God through Jesus Christ. Once this bond is activated, it reflects the highest quality of our human purpose and the greatest mark of our faith in God.

Concepts regarding God's omnipotence and being born again represent two of many areas commonly confused by misconceptions. The situation is significant enough that players, in providing clarification on biblical points, must guard against futile attempts. In some instances, trying to blend physical reality with a spiritual

102

concept can be as difficult as mixing oil and water. Ending up with two broken cheekbones by turning the other cheek too many times is not the desired effect of loving our enemies.[64]

Worse than misplaying our faith is performing in the game with a "faith handicap." Handicapped players have little more than excuses, fears, and doubts to contribute to the game. Moreover, they will grab a wooden nickel in a minute.

Playing the game of life with minimal faith is acceptable to God. However, choosing this level of performance is risky because we are more likely to contaminate our purpose than stay the course of faith. Our pursuits in life are likely to become less God-based and more self-based. Self-based players are far more physical than spiritual. This assertion holds for any population of players.

For the sake of expressing fair kindness with respect to social rejects, many of these players are probably half physical and half spiritual. Some of them, from serial killers and rapists to pathological liars, are the first to acknowledge their faith in God, thereby distinguishing themselves from atheists.

Limiting ourselves to the quality of a physical player does, however, closely align us with atheists. A significant difference is who calls whom in times of trouble. Pending the seriousness of their situations, physical players and atheists normally have the unmitigated gall to call on God without hesitation, though physical players are more likely to make on-the-spot promises to God just to gain His favor. Regardless of how critical moments turn out, physical players are probably quicker in resuming old habits. Meanwhile, atheists primarily need an indisputable and personal show of God's hand to make them believers. Once they are able to declare for themselves what God does and can absorb the wonders of His works, some apply for home team membership. Whenever this kind of conversion takes place, God is ecstatic!

Whereas the best of faithful players have weak moments, the worst of physical players are addicted to doing wrong. They have greater consistency as bigamists in the game because their faith is severely handicapped. Instead of building a relationship with God that keeps Him centrally located in their lives, the weakest and most physical of players constantly cheat on God. They engage in long-term extra-physical affairs of the heart and mind.

While hell may not have the fury of a woman scorned, it houses the souls of many players who, because of God's fury, were rejected at the finish line. These would be the souls of players who never managed to "get set" properly for the race of life because they constantly chose ungodly marks throughout the game. Next to this situation are players who waste opportunities to repent. The most regrettable consequence of this action is not reaching God in time to make the cut for heaven.

Getting set is about as "ready" as we will ever be in the game. Some of the slowest people on earth can get into heaven much quicker or at the same rate of speed as the fastest of players because they primarily stay set throughout the game. This is the most advanced level of performance that players can achieve in the game. Since there is always something for us to do by way of repenting for our sins, staying set is also the best position for us to be in. Besides, the race of life is not won by swiftness; neither is it won by a show of mental greatness.

In the spiritual sense of life, winning is always a matter of our personal faith in God. By choice, we can run the entire race of life without faith. But at some time during the race, players **must** run with a degree of faith just to be considered for the crown of eternal life. This requirement is an unconditional standard for our performance in the game.

Actual attainment of the crown is God's call to make and depends on how we either exercise or fail to exercise faith in God. The race gets tough under both circumstances and, in both cases, many players respond with the same behavior. Regardless of how much God wants us to rely on Him or how much we trust Him to deliver us from the ruts of life, some of us become spiritually disoriented and tumble from the mark of faith.

When faced with critical situations, falling into instant traps of pouting, doubting, and questioning or blaming God for our misfortunes is almost typical behavior. These instinctive binges of behavior happen among the strongest as well as the weakest of believers. In some critical situations, players are also known to flood God with a slew of selfish demands and bargains. Worse than these reactions, some players actually desert God, forgetting that He is the main power switch to our supply of air, heat, and water.

Overall, these responses to God are careless moves in the game that can easily alter our mark and defeat our purpose. They expose us running the race with a clogged faith that yields to bitterness, doubt, and fear. Such a display of faith is an insult to God. Whether either of these responses is temporary or permanent, they compromise the power of faith and show a lack of spiritual wisdom. While the manual reveals that we can do all these things through Christ, who strengthens us, this concept is also one that requires common sense.[65]

For reasons that the least faithful of players can understand as much as any other player, God is not about to strengthen us to always have our way in life. Many times, because of our undermining tendencies, God's discretion in responding to us is the main factor in the game that protects us from our own actions. In response to His intervening nature, we should be eager to just show Him our appreciation.

We should also be grateful that our every wish is not granted because a few players bypass the sanity of faith altogether. The more critical their circumstances, the more irrational they are in their spiritual behavior. When a loved one dies, for example, to pray for that person's return to life is an extreme misuse of faith, but not because this would be an impossible task for God. He has done far more incredible things and remains in the miracle business all day, every day. Even so, the last miracle of resurrection took place so long ago that in these modern times, anybody returning days later from the dead would probably scare onlookers to death. This kind of fear is best left in reserve for more practical matters, such as the possibility of spending eternity in hell.

However extreme this case may be, it promotes the need for us to exercise faith with spiritual maturity. Only in this fashion are we capable of becoming effective managers of life. Spiritual maturity puts us in the best position to accept and deal with the harsh inevitabilities of life that we wish were different and, in some cases, totally avoidable.

In situations of disappointment, grief, illness, and other major upsets in life, faith is our power tool for survival. As the height of spiritual maturity, faith enables us to understand that reliance on God does not free us of tough circumstances. Many times when we seek God's relief, His response may not be immediate by human stan-

106

dards. But, while relief is on the way, God strengthens us through our faith to endure the wait.

At any given time, more players than not have probably prayed earnestly for the same help, but failed to receive the same response from God. There are also times when God just outright denies our requests, and not because they are necessarily ill-intended or senseless. As our Father, He has the parental right to reject our petitions; besides, saying no is what many parents do best.

Contrary to the beliefs of some players, when God denies our wishes, he is not ignoring us. He is simply taking care of His business. His purpose in our lives takes precedence and, therefore, will be executed whether we are pleased or not. Those of us who would abandon God on this basis should reflect immediately on the many times when we disappoint God because of choices that we make. Fortunately, in view of His jealous nature, He never pays us back by forsaking us. Otherwise, we would not have a lifetime of chances to kiss and make up and to mess up again; yet, so many of us do not take advantage of this generous God-given provision.

Sometimes, God rejects our requests for our own good; at other times, the situation could be that He has something else in store for us. Whatever His reasons are, our purpose in the game is to never doubt His faithfulness to us and to trust His love as the personal foundation of our lives.

A cherished friend of mine, the late Reverend Carzell Reid, often expressed his faith with this sobering thought: "I rather believe that it is a hell and find out that it's not, than believe that it is not a hell and find out that it is." As a closing point on this segment of playing the game of life, players are much better off believing God is and finding out that He's not, than believing God is not and finding out that He is.

Ultimately, our faith in God measures our love for Him and our hope to wear the crown of eternal life.

Leap for Joy! (Strategic Foundations of the Game)

Hearts, minds, and egos are basic muscles of human pursuits. They can enhance our performance and propel us to great heights of joy or deaden our efforts and, with the same ease, drive us into the deepest pits of despair. In the absence of personal ambition, we may also be left to wallow in fields of mediocrity. Either way, with God's impending forecast for our lives, our every move in the game hinges on the mandates of these muscles. These tendencies are confirmed standards of the game.

More than other human features in the game, our hearts, minds, and egos are directly responsible for the quality of our obedience to God. With the exception of God's power, they have the most immediate influence on the energy and level of commitment with which we pursue the primary goal of the game and our personal missions in life.

These same three features are also the greatest source of spiritual interference. They constantly interrupt the balance of our faith and deeds. At times, some home team players are thrown completely off their mark of faith. The further we land from our point of balance, the more urgent our need is to reestablish a mark of faith; we need to **get set** again.

In some situations, the urgency of getting set again requires building anew our relationship with God. In the case of players who have deliberately been away from church for a significant while, reinstatement of membership is imperative. The general need in other cases is probably a matter of spiritual proficiency. We must always strive to be spiritually alert and skilled enough to combat the moves of Satan and his team.

More importantly, we must remember that Satan's only aim on earth is to gain full control over all of God's properties. His main prop in this effort is an updated file that he always maintains on the home team. He carefully studies the habits and playing styles of all members, whether they have pledged lifetime commitment to the team or not. The total scope of his preoccupation with recruiting players from God's team involves many schemes. His most notorious routine is hanging around in their midst as he does with all other players, and for as long as he can without much concern about being discovered.

Despite any credits due for his success on the playing fields of life, the devil is far from ever becoming victorious. His experience of being avoided and having his appeals refused is much too great. More than any player in the game, the devil is quite aware of his limitations and realizes that he will never be forceful enough to put God, nor any of God's key players, out of business. Though his lifetime record of isolation and rejections has already proven this situation to be true, failure is his primary source of motivation. Accordingly, he will never give up his obsessive determination to rid God of His supreme nature and dominance. Otherwise, most of his time would not be spent learning how to best disguise himself as a home team player.

However slick the devil may be in attempts to contaminate the human experience, the strongest of home team players will always be his worst nightmare.

Every player needs a master plan of faith. The game of life is all about winning, and winning is all about having faith. In this respect, faith is a way of life that demands our focus on God as a means of promoting His cause on earth. This level of commitment to God goes beyond resisting the devil, but does not ignore the belief that his stalking presence in the game will always require our vigilance. On any day, while roaming among God's flock, he alternates his attire between sheep and wolves' clothing, pretending to be one thing and, then, another.

Besides the devil's modes of distraction, players are challenged by a number of personal matters that include marriage and divorce, careers, finances, church and health issues, friendships, and self-image. Over time, these matters can escalate into situations that are stressful enough to test the strongest of faithful players.

Given these situations and all other factors that influence our lives, change is probably the most prominent because it challenges our faith about as much as the devil does. The immediate effect impacts our performance as a spice; either it's too much, just right, or not enough. Seldom is change just right because nothing in life stays the same. The natural force of change separates men from boys, women from girls, and effective managers of life from those of us who simply exist day by day.

All that we do in life is accompanied by change because change comes with **the turf.** It comes with the birth and death of each player as it does with the dawn and sunset of each day. We change with every breath that we take. Regardless of how carefully we plan our lives, change is an inconvenience as much as it is convenience. A shattering example is losing one dentist to retirement

111

and searching for another who has the same quality of skills and care.

As the bearer of all things known and unknown in life, change presents us with possibilities that spread our options between the positive and negative extremities of life.

The composite record of human experience and time shows that selfish and other unkind pursuits usually result in personal losses instead of gains. In the highest dimension of the game, we risk much more than material possessions when we consciously choose to align our moral allegiance with doctrines, rules, and practices that conflict with God. A double risk occurs when we consistently submit to the ways of Satan because we also jeopardize our souls.

Unfortunately, the value of these age-old cautions has never stopped players from burying their heads in the sand. Human nature makes us gullible to the extent that taking chances is normal in the game. Yet, because of the difference in our personal allegiance, many of us withstand the temptation of making choices that we know will have harmful effects on our lives. This difference is why some of us choose to build and share our resources for the common good of mankind, rather than restrict our energies to keeping up with the Jones family. For reasons already implied, players differ on the image that they wish to project.

In the natural course of the game, we all change for the better or we change for the worse. Whether change is quick, slow, or sneaky, there is very little about the human experience that does not change. This condition is the pure nature of the game. After all, change is the stuff of life that builds up the good old days. In fact, if it were not for change, players would never stand a chance of getting into heaven. Lest we forget, change is the ultimate declaration of faith and the process by which all players get set for the race of life.

From a strategic point of view, we cannot isolate our faith as a secret weapon to be drawn in times of distress. Any concealment of faith lessens our spiritual sight on God and further minimizes our reverence for Him.

Inasmuch as players do not have full access to God's plan of action, we will never know or understand everything about Him. This does not mean that God is a big secret to be kept in the game. Neither is He some monumental mystery to be solved; He just happens to move in a way that is mysterious to us.[66]

The fact that we do not know everything about God and His plans makes faith all the more crucial to our performance. It causes our success to be totally dependent upon our willingness to believe in Him with due respect for His privacy, and to stand in awe of all the many wonders performed by His mighty power.

Believing in God with gratitude and a profound commitment to serve Him is our unchanging purpose in the game. Furthermore, as undeserving subjects of His love and faithfulness, our bounding duty is to proclaim His glory as much as we can. Most of all, we should never put God in the position of relying on rocks to do our job. This kind of performance is the worst display of spiritual negligence and the worst way to lose the game. Therefore, we should praise Him for as long as we have the health and strength to do so.

Faith is our most vital link to the purpose, plan, and process that God has to accommodate us in His spirit. Strategically, we cannot afford anything less than an enduring faith to accommodate Him in our lives.

Every player should know the ABCs of wor-

ship. Christmas is a time of year that always seems to make the world a better place. It binds the greatest number of players to the common cause of remembering God's greatest love offering to the world, that being Jesus Christ. In addition to inciting the traditional hype of last-minute shopping, the spirit of Christmas lifts us to levels of arresting hatred and releasing love for almost twenty-four hours.

By our actions, this long-awaited and special pause in the game does little more than reduce Christmas Day to being another Sunday of the year; after Sunday, Monday always comes. Likewise, very early in the aftermath of Christmas Day, the cluttered trenches of life demand our immediate return to active duty. Somehow, through the fading glee and glitter of the season, the unpleasant stings of life are also resumed. What a sad commentary it is that we allow our commemoration of the most blessed event known to be so temporary!

The love that endears us to one another while we celebrate the birth of Christ is becoming ever so brief. More critical than the growing brevity of that love is the interval of our behavior from one Christmas Day to the next. During the eagerness of our natural retreat to the best and worst of times, players also return to their good, bad, and ugly ways of life. In the process, Jesus continues to be crucified about as much as He is adored.

However righteous or sinful our behavior may be, the Christmas season holds no monopoly on motivating players to a time of worship. In conjunction with our common purpose in the game, worship is a routine expression of faith. Ordinarily, worship is a function of our circumstances, desires, fulfillments, and spiritual responsibilities, but the quality of our worship is determined by our individual character.

Physical players are basically impassionate in their worship; their motive is to please the public or to secure their public image. Though spiritual players are more committed worshipers, they are also flawed with impassionate tendencies. Players of both groups are accustomed to saying "Thank you, Lord!" or "Oh my God!" without any forethought of worship. Outside the realm of worship, these dramatic remarks are generally spoken to bring closure on situations that are the least expected. Players who escape going to jail because of a technicality thank God just as quickly and easily as many players do when their children *finally* graduate from high school.

In yet another situation that's altogether different, perhaps the most inciting comment is, "Thank God it's Friday!"

As a genuine expression of faith, worship has a much greater value of inducing a "spiritual high." The impact relieves the pressure of whatever ails us and soothes us when we are not ailing at all. Beyond having a cure-all effect, worship is the primary means of praising the God whom we celebrate as Creator and Father of mankind.

In accordance with religious customs practiced by cultures of their respective generation, players have always worshiped a deity of some kind. Of the many gods served in ancient times and through the present day, only one God has been everlasting from the beginning of time. This only God was the God of Abraham and Moses, and the only God equipped with a love broad enough to save the whole world from sin. This same God is the only God who abides with us as the Holy Spirit of Jesus Christ; He rules the world and "is worthy to be praised."[67]

Whether in a public or private setting, the experience of worship is a three-in-one opportunity for players to engage in personal communion with God. One of the fulfilling components of this experience is music. Players have been encouraged through the ages to "sing unto the Lord."[68] As a tactful reminder for those of us who are not endowed with such talent, humming unto the Lord is probably just as pleasing to His ears. Maybe, for the comfort of others who happen to be around, the best choice would be listening while they sing. Clapping to the beat works just as well, depending on our location at the time.

An option worthy of serious consideration is writing lyrics for others to sing. Many anthems, gospel songs, and hymns are adaptations from the Old Testament of the Bible. Several of those that are currently sung in worship services or by recording artists are based on the **Psalms of David:** O Lord, How Excellent (8); The Lord Is My Shepherd (23); The Lord is My Light and My Salvation (27); O Rest in the Lord (37); Bless the Lord, O my Soul (103); and, If It Had Not Been for the Lord on My Side (124).

Songs of faith enhance our spiritual growth and game performance in a number of significant ways. They contain messages of worship that reflect our personal needs, define our relationship to God, and declare commitments of faith between God and man. On a more personal level, the lyrics of these songs affirm God's provisions of assurance, consolation, hope, joy, peace, and strength. The realness of these offerings constantly broadens our perspective of the glory of God. Hence, to sing unto the Lord is to glorify Him in the highest; to worship Him is to magnify His prominence in all the earth.

The value of prayer and reading the Holy Scriptures matches the value of music as primary means of worship. Each of these emphases complements the remaining two. Music is often a background prop for prayers; some worship groups sing awhile and pray awhile; and Scriptures are incorporated in prayers as much as they are in the lyrics of some songs.

Players are able to receive the same basic benefits from musical, prayerful, and Scriptural contacts with God. Our spirits are lifted by either source, but each of these three components of worship engages us in a different way.

Sacred music has a way of instantly transforming our mental or emotional state into a happier presence of mind. Even the physically impaired and spiritually lame have cause to leap for joy. Upon occasions, if only for one moment, this music also stimulates the moral conscience of our soul. Prayer and biblical Scriptures go a bit further in this gratifying experience and, therefore, impact our performance in other ways.

Prayer takes us into a deeper and more personalized dimension of worship, and varies according to our circumstances at the time. One minute, it's a two-word distress signal to God when we need Him to get us out of trouble as soon as *yesterday*. At other times, it is an expression of gratitude to thank Him for bringing us through rough periods of disappointment, pain, grief, loss, and other woes. There are also times when prayer is a prolonged list of the many situations that we want God to fix in His own time, but not necessarily in His own way.

A close examination of the Lord's Prayer makes it plain that several objectives are to be achieved when we "routinely" approach God in prayer:[69]

1. We should acknowledge His existence and position of authority in the game. ("Our Father . . .")
2. We should exalt His presence. ("Hallowed be thy name.")

3. We should submit ourselves to His purpose. ("Thy will be done in earth. . . .")
4. We should seek His love and grace. ("Give us this day our daily bread.")
5. We should humble ourselves unto His mercy. ("Forgive us our debts. . . .")
6. We should rely on His counsel and His assuring arm of defense. ("Lead us not into temptation, but deliver us from evil. . . .")
7. We should celebrate His omnipotent presence and proclaim His absolute dominion over all things. ("For thine is the kingdom, and the power, and the glory, for ever. Amen.")

The Bible is also an unchanging and irreplaceable source of worship. In modern day practices of organized religion, we are adjusting to a shift from conventional hymns to contemporary songs of faith. Other efforts to modernize worship include contemporary performances in dance and drama. Whether these moves prove to be long-standing or not, they will never overshadow the significance of the Holy Scriptures as an aspect of worship.

Aside from being an ample source of inspiration, the Bible is the pervasive organ of God that calls all players to worship Him: "O come, let us worship and bow down: let us kneel before the Lord our maker."[70] This summons refines the field of our responsibilities to God. It also directs the trail of our faith in God.

Summarily, sacred music, prayer, and the Holy Scriptures are primary components of the Christian faith through which we engage ourselves in worship. The summons for us to worship and bow down before God automatically dismisses worship as an optional exercise of faith. In fact, David proceeds with worship as an all inclusive mandate: "Let every thing that hath breath praise the Lord."[71]

While pursuing the ultimate reward of faith, the toast from our hearts should be equally compelling:

> Here's looking to you, God; our help in ages gone by and our hope in coming years. We worship you in the name of your Son, Jesus Christ, in whom you have entrusted all power to present us faultless before your throne. AMEN.

Every player has a designated position in the game. All of us are not avid sports fans, and some sports enthusiasts do not like all sports. Neither do they attend or watch sporting events for the same reasons. The only purpose may be to support and encourage a relative or friend who is a participant. Sometimes, as the case is with gatherings at homecoming games and annual Super Bowl parties, several of those in attendance know absolutely nothing about football and could care less about who wins. Their main objective is to eat, drink, and be merry.

Such an event may be a first-time experience that bores some people to the extent of wishing that they had not come. Pending the nature of an event, leaving before it's over can be more of a disadvantage than staying. Unless an emergency occurs, sometimes leaving early is an insult.

In other cases, watching televised sports or engaging in something else may be the only thing that appeals at the time. After all, as it is with many things that we randomly do—whether harmless or harmful—watching television is a way of passing the time of day.

These situations briefly describe patterns of how we actually play the game of life. Unfortunately, everybody is not enthusiastic about playing the game. Some of us would prefer leaving before our playing time is up, but remain because of the alternative. Under the most depressive of circumstances, players are quite aware that the only way to leave the game voluntarily is by way of suicide. With such a critical and final choice to make, players who either fear bumbling their efforts in such a drastic step or have no zest for life usually choose to stay in the game as passive participants. Several resort to living in seclusion or as a hobo.

More often than not, we slip, fall, and slip or fall again because of our steps and missteps in life. While fumbling around on our feet is par course for the game, having a sense of direction is altogether different. Our chosen course in life measures the quality of our maturity and the strength of our faith. The longer our strides, the further we may go; and the steadier our strides, the more likely we are to reach our destination on earth. The quality of our game rests, therefore, with where we plan to go and how we intend to get there.

Our major and minor steps in the game are based on the kind of character that we develop over time through personal experiences. The lot of this development includes faith, self-esteem, interests, skills, and sportsmanship. This notion accounts for the purpose of formal education and systems of religion. It is also a reason for parents to involve their children in piano and dance lessons and little league sports.

Early training is expected to get us ahead in some intervals of the game, but progressive training is more profitable in making us better prepared to play the game. Either way, the gains acquired from these provisions should benefit our missions on earth and our goal after death. The more prepared we are for the world of work, the better our chances are for being hired. By the same logic, the more prepared we are for the kingdom of heaven, the better our chances are for spending eternity with God.

Whether we are focused on the here and now or the "there and then" of our future, the Bible is a complete guide for our preparations. It is the multi-purpose textbook of faith that offers the best strategic plan for securing our present and future life on earth and our hope of eternal rest.

The first point of this plan is, perhaps, the most obvious in presenting God's position on the brotherhood of man. It confirms the lyrics, "No man is an island," and implicates God's use of Adam's rib to create woman. The supposition is simple.

If God had intended for man to live alone, we would be playing on His turf at the human rate of one person at a time. Even in our wildest imagination, the reality of one person living on earth in today's world is difficult to conceive.

Due to God's executive decision, the game of life is the only individual sport that man has no possibility of playing alone. Before his death, Howard Hughes, a public figure of wealth and clout, was an example of proof. His billions of dollars could not afford him exclusive rights to pure seclusion. If for no other reason, he was reduced to relying on servants and doctors for physical comfort.

People of lesser means who are not totally dependent on welfare assistance are neither totally self-supporting. Yet, some of them also prefer living in seclusion. Seldom do they realize that God is responsible for the person who invented the machinery from whence their pay checks are mechanically produced.

God administers to us on a daily basis through professionals in all walks of life. So, for those of us who recognize God as the only benefactor needed in life, common sense adds another perspective. God is all that we will ever need, and we need Him in every form that He avails Himself to us.

While none of us chose to be born, each of us is involved with a world of all kinds of people. According to the plan, we must learn to effectively manage hatred and bigotry, serve the sick and needy, and create a climate to tolerate different opinions, values, attitudes, and customs. At the same time, our sinful ways must be handled with a firm hand of compassion and discipline. In the truest sense of brotherhood, we must also learn to love our neighbors and our enemies.[72]

Another point of the plan requires us to share our talents. Regardless of whether they are hidden or not, we can be sure that every player has at least one. They are the inner fruit of our bodies used by God to satisfy the will of His purpose, even when that purpose is to make somebody smile.

Our talents are also means by which God shows us the right and wrong ways of life and related consequences. As it is with most of what we do in life, God allows us the choice of using our talents as we see fit. We can either follow the example of a servant who buried his opportunity in life, or take the way of two other servants who doubled their opportunities.[73] There are no restrictions on how much we share of ourselves, neither is there an age limit.

In recent years, our nation applauded the generous spirit of Alexandra Scott, a young cancer victim who died at the age of eight in 2004. During her brief lifetime, this young Philadelphian inspired lemonade stands throughout the United States and Canada that grossed almost a million dollars to aid pediatric cancer research. Another young victim, Mattie Stepanek, who lost his battle with Muscular Dystrophy in the same year, charmed the world with his insatiable passion for life and writing. In response to the bravery that he demonstrated in his plight, Mattie was appointed National Goodwill Ambassador for the Muscular Dystrophy Association.

Essentially, our pursuits on earth are part mission and part ministry. Our performance in each dimension should be personally fulfilling, but when we freely use what God endows us with for the benefit of others, our pursuits become "faith-filling" ministries.

On a practical level, our ministries establish our playing position in the game; they are the "knacks" that we have in life. Some are natural; some are not. Babies have an inborn knack for crying while their parents develop a series of knacks for quieting them.

That explanation makes it plain that our ministries are not necessarily connected to a line of work. Any number of players have a knack for making people happy, and some others have a knack for getting on everybody's last nerve.

Whether we have a knack for sewing, concocting recipes, gardening, or doing other things, the desire to share the fruit of our labors enhances the quality of our performance.

Our position in the game varies according to the play period, social needs and circumstances, and the span of our effectiveness. We tend to rely on others because they have the best reputation for doing whatever it is that they do best. Players often rise to administrative positions because they have a knack for leadership and resolving problems. Every so often, however, we are unsuccessful in our ministries.

During a conference of professional school counselors

that I attended, one of the keynote speakers talked of a man standing on a bridge with the intention of committing suicide. Along came a counselor, well-regarded for the success of his people skills and handling crises. He eventually coaxed the troubled man from the bridge and counseled him. Minutes later, they both jumped.

The implications of this tale are several. Most important to our performance is realizing our limitations. We are not able to be all things to all people simply because we do not perform well in all areas of life. Usually, a bowler is not expected to have the skills of an opera singer, nor is an opera singer expected to have skills comparable to those of an astronaut. And, yet, stranger things are possible.

Knacks are also true expressions of character. They create consistency in our behavior and cause our responses to be predictable in most situations. This thought points to the image of players who have a knack for being objective and of godly principles. Instead of sitting idly by in the midst of wrongdoing, these players are known to stand for right even if they must stand alone. Knacks of this kind have merit in the game as strategic moves of obedience to God.[74]

Regardless of the position by which we are identified in the game, having a knack for getting God's undivided attention is the most natural talent that any player develops. Sharing this particular art of "hooking up" with God is the **final point of strategy.** Success with this part of the plan is a matter of attitude.

The world, with all of its diversity and adversity, is actually a beautiful place to be. However, one exception prevails. We seem to take a step backward on all the fronts of life. The most disturbing matter regarding this plight is the continued debate of "creation versus evolution." Given our sinful ways and all that God has brought us through, seemingly, we would be more solid in our position on this matter. Instead, Bible battles are taking us further from being one nation under God to becoming a nation without any particular claim to faith. After centuries of attending church, we are a "churched" people who still doubt the authenticity of God's position in the game. On the other hand, however, we are also becoming an "unchurched" people who believe in God.

Neither of these extremes has a valid place in the game; nevertheless, the situation is **real** and has an extensive impact on how some players perceive the goal of the game. One of the worst outcomes would be newer standards to further slight God's position in the game. In the case of such newness, chances are "God" would be stricken from the print of our patriotic songs and customary utterances of "God bless America" would be prohibited by law.

Indeed, we are experiencing trying times that test our souls to the quick; but we are also living in the presence of hope. God has already ordered a time when wickedness shall cease and the weary shall rest.[75] In the interest of preserving spiritual dignity, our position should be in compliance with the command that urges "men ought always to pray, and not to faint."[76] Inasmuch as Jesus cited the command, prayer has to be a sure way of getting God's attention.

At best, prayer assures us that God is the same today as on yesterday and tomorrow; and, until the end of time, He is also the Alpha and Omega of life.[77] Just as He knows our needs before we ask, He naturally knew our position in life before our birth. However, what God wants from us is another matter. Regardless of our character and behavior, casting our cares on God means more

125

to Him than, perhaps, His assurance of grace and mercy means to us.

Meanwhile, in the run of social change, the church on the street corner may fail, but the spiritual establishment of God will not. Educational and governmental services may shut down, but god's hand of relief will not. Marriage and family life may dissolve, but God's covenant will not. The emphasis of brotherhood may be weakened by modern technology, but our union with God will not.

Ultimately, the opposition will be defeated and the home team will soar to the throne of God through victory in Jesus Christ. Those among us who wish to take that journey are reminded of the need to follow the strategic commands of God:

1. Seek ye first the kingdom of heaven (Matthew 6:33).
2. Trust in the Lord with all thine heart; and lean not unto thine own understanding. In all thy ways acknowledge Him (Proverbs 3:5–6).
3. Look to the hills from whence your help comes (Psalm 121:1).
4. Ask, and it shall be given you; seek, and ye shall find; knock, and it shall be opened unto you (Matthew 7:7).
5. Wait on the Lord (Psalm 27:14).
6. Be strong and take courage (Joshua 1:6).
7. Get wisdom and understanding (Proverbs 4:7).
8. Shun evil; do good and seek peace (1 Peter 3:11).

Many of our misplays in the history of the game are not erasable, but they can be corrected. Mahatma Gandhi, Dr. Martin Luther King, Jr., and Mother Teresa are among primary honorees whom we recognize for their efforts in making the world a better place and the game of life a better sport. There are also millions of unsung heroes and trench soldiers who are equally important. Unfortunately, the battles that they fought are still being fought.

We have come too far in the game as a world, nation, and as individuals to be so far behind in our focus and values. While a few players in the game are ahead of "the boat," too few are playing in the boat. Many of those playing behind cannot find the boat because they do not have a knack for believing in God; hence, they have neither the will nor the vision needed for pursuing God's purpose.

The beauty of staying the course with God until we reach the finish line is earning the right to claim Paul's position: "I have fought a good fight, I have finished my course, I have kept the faith."[78] Actual achievement of that position may be our only pass into the kingdom of heaven. Perchance we reach the gates, what a great and endless joy God's welcoming voice must be: **"Well done, my good and faithful servant!"**

Believe Now, Fly Later!
(The Final Beginning)

The social forecast for tomorrow's world includes showers of moderate to rapid change with sudden floods of turbulence, but the game of life will continue according to schedule. As a means of maintaining high level visibility, players are urged to proceed with consistency in faith, hope, and love.

Eventually, Santa Claus and the tooth fairy may be dismissed as dignitaries of childhood, but God will always rule the world as the "Chief Dignitary" of life and the human experience. Regardless of our many playing errors, God will also remain a public force of love, grace, and mercy.

From this point, further coverage on the game is impossible because God declares all winners and losers after their final breath on earth. Since the next phase of the game starts in eternity, the summary of this entire presentation begins with comments on the chambers that await our souls.

Heaven and hell are two places in eternity yet unseen by human eyes, but both dimensions are physical realities of faith. After riding the transport of life on earth, each player spends eternity in only one of these two places. The ride is a one-time adventure that unfolds as the most unique sport ever played by humankind; it is a woman and man's game and the game of every child.

Since heaven is God's home, it is the sky-mansion where the souls of His champions gather for eternal rest. Getting to this resting place is the earth-while goal of human pursuit. **On God's Turf** presents greater coverage on going to heaven because heaven is believed to be the most desired destination of man.

The game of life has been covered as a special interest sport produced, sponsored, and managed by God as an opportunity for all players to prove their worthiness for heaven. Anybody who accepts the challenge is required to believe in **The Holy Trinity** of God the Father, Son, and Holy Spirit. God's position of authority must also be recognized as the only feature in the equation of human existence that has ultimate control over the present, future, and final course of our lives.

Our best show of allegiance to God is living according to **His Word** as recorded in the Holy Bible. This commitment binds us to a "Believe now, fly later" plan of faith in Jesus Christ.

Fighting constant battles between good and evil while contending with other rough spots in the game is not easy, but survival is always possible when we play by faith. An enduring faith is but one tool of stability that enables us to absorb ourselves in the presence of God and the reality of His perfection. In the process, we learn that the game is not really about our purpose as much as it is about God's purpose in our lives. Better still, the game is about God's covenant with all players, whether we ignore or seek to do His will. The ideal agenda is to be constantly transformed from who and where we are to who we want to become and where we want to go in the spirit of Jesus Christ.

While Earth remains the feeder planet to heaven and hell, the game of life will continue as a sport designed by

God for every player that has breath. Conclusively, the God celebrated in the Players' Manual as Creator, Owner, and Sustainer of life reserves all rights to the game and to each past, present, and future player. These are the terms for playing on His turf, whether in a state of allegiance to Him or to Satan; henceforth and forever. AMEN.

Scriptural References (All Biblical Notations Are Based on the King James Version of the Holy Bible.)

1. Exodus 20:3–7
2. Mark 11:25–26
3. Deuteronomy 32:4
4. Isaiah 7:14
5. John 14:6
6. John 3:15–16
7. Matthew 4:17
8. Matthew 7:21
9. James 2:26
10. Psalm 24:1
11. Psalm 100:3
12. Matthew 16:18
13. Romans 3:23
14. Ephesians 6:11
15. Matthew 17:20
16. 2 Timothy 1:7
17. 1 Corinthians 13:13
18. Proverbs 22:6
19. Philippians 4:19
20. Mark 4:39
21. 1 Corinthians 13:11
22. Matthew 6:19–21
23. Mark 8:36
24. Ezekiel 18:30
25. Matthew 5:16
26. Proverbs 15:1
27. Luke 19:40
28. Isaiah 40:31
29. 1 Corinthians 13:12
30. See Supplementary References
31. Leviticus 18:22
32. Isaiah 2:4
33. Ecclesiastes 3:8
34. Isaiah 9:6
35. Matthew 5:9
36. Proverbs 3:6
37. Matthew 22:39
38. Matthew 26:39, 42
39. Matthew 7:7–8
40. Matthew 16:18
41. See Supplementary References
42. See Supplementary References
43. Ephesians 1:22–23
44. Matthew 24:36, 42; 25:13
45. Deuteronomy 26:18
46. Psalm 37:7
47. Genesis 9:1
48. Genesis 3:1–6
49. Job 2:9
50. Genesis 1:26–27
51. Psalm 8:5; Isaiah 55:8
52. Genesis 1:28
53. Galatians 6–9
54. Genesis 6:14–16, 7:4
55. Matthew 26:22
56. Matthew 26:69–75
57. John 20:24–29
58. Matthew 5:3–10
59. John 3:15–16
60. Luke 23:39–43
61. Exodus 20:5
62. John 3:1–5
63. Matthew 14:17–21
64. Matthew 5:39
65. Philippians 4:13
66. Mark 4:22; Luke 12:8–9
67. Psalm 18:3
68. Exodus 15:21
69. Matthew 6:9–13
70. Psalm 95:6
71. Psalm 150:6

72. Matthew 5:43–44
73. Matthew 25:15–29
74. Leviticus 5:1
75. Job 3:17
76. Luke 18:1
77. Revelations 1:8
78. 2 Timothy 4:7

Supplementary References

30. *Brown v. Board of Education of Topeka.* 347 U.S. 483, 74 S.Ct. 686, 98 L. Ed. 873 (1954).
41. Palmer, R. R. *A History of the Modern World* (New York: Alfred A. Knopf, 1959) pp. 21–78.
42. Ibid., p. 78.